Identity Construction and Illness Narratives in Persons with Disabilities

This book investigates how being diagnosed with various disabilities impacts on identity. Once diagnosed with a disability, there is a risk that this label can become the primary status both for the person diagnosed as well as for their family. This reification of the diagnosis can be oppressive because it subjugates humanity in such a way that everything a person does can be interpreted as linked to their disability.

Drawing on narrative approaches to identity in psychology and social sciences, the bio-psycho-social model and a holistic approach to disabilities, the chapters in this book understand disability as constructed in discourse, as negotiated among speaking subjects in social contexts, and as emergent. By doing so, they amplify voices that may have otherwise remained silent and use storytelling as a way of communicating the participants' realities to provide a more in-depth understanding of their point of view.

This book will be of interest to all scholars and students of disability studies, sociology, medical humanities, disability research methods, narrative theory, and rehabilitation studies.

Chalotte Glintborg is a scientist from Aalborg University, Denmark, who specializes in rehabilitation psychology and holds a PhD in psychology. Her research has centred on exploring first-person perspectives on the emotional consequences of living with illness/disabilities, e.g. identity problems, distress, shame, and depression, etc.

Manuel L. de la Mata is full professor in the Department of Experimental Psychology at the University of Seville, Spain, and the head of the Laboratory of Human Activity Research Group and holds a PhD in psychology. His recent research has centred on the narrative construction of self and autobiographical memory in cultural context, and gender and culture.

Interdisciplinary Disability Studies

Series editor: Mark Sherry, The University of Toledo, USA

Disability studies has made great strides in exploring power and the body. This series extends the interdisciplinary dialogue between disability studies and other fields by asking how disability studies can influence a particular field. It will show how a deep engagement with disability studies changes our understanding of the following fields: sociology, literary studies, gender studies, bioethics, social work, law, education, or history. This ground-breaking series identifies both the practical and theoretical implications of such an interdisciplinary dialogue and challenges people in disability studies as well as other disciplinary fields to critically reflect on their professional praxis in terms of theory, practice, and methods.

Critical Disability Studies and the Disabled Child
Unsettling Distinctions
Harriet Cooper

Disability, Globalization and Human Rights
Edited by Hisayo Katsui and Shuaib Chalklen

Reimagining Disablist and Ableist Violence as Abjection
Ryan Thorneycroft

Identity Construction and Illness Narratives in Persons with Disabilities
Chalotte Glintborg and Manuel L. de la Mata

Disability and Citizenship Studies
Marie Sépulchre

Women with Disabilities as Agents of Peace, Change and Rights
Experiences from Sri Lanka
Edited by Karen Soldatic and Dinesha Samararatne

For a full list of titles in this series, please visit: www.routledge.com/series/ASHSER1401

Identity Construction and Illness Narratives in Persons with Disabilities

Edited by
Chalotte Glintborg and Manuel L. de la Mata

Routledge
Taylor & Francis Group
LONDON AND NEW YORK

First published 2021
by Routledge
2 Park Square, Milton Park, Abingdon, Oxon OX14 4RN

and by Routledge
605 Third Avenue, New York, NY 10017

First issued in paperback 2022

Routledge is an imprint of the Taylor & Francis Group, an informa business

Publisher's Note
The publisher has gone to great lengths to ensure the quality of this reprint but points out that some imperfections in the original copies may be apparent.

British Library Cataloguing-in-Publication Data
A catalogue record for this book is available from the British Library

Library of Congress Cataloging-in-Publication Data
Names: Glintborg, Chalotte, editor. | Mata, Manuel de la, 1961- editor.
Title: Identity construction and illness narratives in persons with disabilities / edited by Chalotte Glintborg and Manuel de la Mata.
Description: Abingdon, Oxon ; New York, NY : Routledge, 2021. | Series: Interdisciplinary disability studies | Includes bibliographical references and index.
Identifiers: LCCN 2020013236 (print) | LCCN 2020013237 (ebook) | ISBN 9780367898717 (hardback) | ISBN 9781003021612 (ebook)
Subjects: LCSH: People with disabilities--Psychology. | Identity (Psychology) | Narrative inquiry (Research method) | Disability studies.
Classification: LCC BF727.P57 .I34 2021 (print) | LCC BF727.P57 (ebook) | DDC 155.9/16--dc23
LC record available at https://lccn.loc.gov/2020013236
LC ebook record available at https://lccn.loc.gov/2020013237

ISBN: 978-0-367-53903-0 (pbk)
ISBN: 978-0-367-89871-7 (hbk)
ISBN: 978-1-003-02161-2 (ebk)

DOI: 10.4324/9781003021612

Typeset in Times New Roman
by Taylor & Francis Books

Contents

Contributors

Nichlas Permin Berger is a researcher at the Danish Center for Social Science Research (VIVE) and part-time lecturer at Aalborg University who specializes in qualitative methods and narrative analysis of vulnerable groups' encounters with welfare state services. He has a PhD in sociology. His research concerns support and treatment, psychiatric diagnoses and identity, risk, responsibilization, and user involvement in social work practices.

Mercedes Cubero is Associate Professor in the Department of Experimental Psychology at the University of Seville, Spain, and a member of the Laboratory of Human Activity Research Group. She has a PhD in psychology. Her recent research has centred on the cultural (re)construction of identity in situations of vulnerability, including women after gender violence, the construction of healthy student identity in contexts of inequality and social exclusion, and identity reconstruction after aphasia.

Rosario Cubero is Associate Professor in the Department of Developmental and Educational Psychology at the University of Seville, Spain, and member of the research group Laboratory of Human Activity. She has a PhD in psychology. Her research has focused on the construction of educational knowledge and the analysis of social interaction in teaching-learning processes. In recent years, she has developed research on the construction of science in higher education, dialogic reflection in teacher training, and the study of learner identity through narratives.

Manuel L. de la Mata is Full Professor in the Department of Experimental Psychology at the University of Seville, Spain, and the head of the Laboratory of Human Activity Research Group and holds a PhD in psychology. His recent research has centred on the narrative construction of self and autobiographical memory in cultural context, and gender and culture.

Mattias Forsblad is a scientist from Linköping University who has specialized in system perspectives on cognition and cognitive ageing in everyday life circumstances for healthy individuals and people with dementia diseases. He has a PhD in cognitive science.

Lars Fynbo is a senior researcher at the Danish Centre for Social Science Research (VIVE) who specializes in qualitative analysis in the alcohol and other drugs research field, and has a PhD in sociology. His research is centred on risk as a social phenomenon and he often applies a user's perspective when investigating risk. He has published research articles about stigmatization processes, risk activities, and qualitative methods.

Chalotte Glintborg is a scientist from Aalborg University, Denmark, who specializes in rehabilitation psychology and holds a PhD in psychology. Her research has centred on exploring first-person perspectives on the emotional consequences of living with illness/disabilities, e.g. identity problems, distress, shame, and depression, etc.

Malin Hallén is a senior lecturer at Halmstad University, Sweden, and has a PhD in media and communication studies. Her research interests include science and health journalism and media representations of health, with a special focus on issues related to mental illness.

Lars-Christer Hydén received his PhD in psychology from the Stockholm University, Sweden. His current position is as professor of social psychology at Linköping University, Sweden, and as director of Center for Dementia Research (CEDER). His research primarily concerns how people with Alzheimer's disease and their significant others interact and use language as a way to sustain and negotiate everyday life and a sense of self.

Kristine Jensen de López is a professor at the Center for Developmental & Applied Psychological Science, Aalborg University, Denmark and has a PhD in developmental psychology. She carries out research on language and communication in typically and atypically developing children, and is director of Aalborg University's children's clinic for developmental communication and language disorders. Related research areas are emotion, social cognition development, and culture.

Rena Lyons is a certified speech and language therapist and senior lecturer in the discipline of speech and language therapy, School of Health Science, College of Medicine, Nursing and Health Science, NUI Galway, Ireland. She has over 30 years of clinical, teaching, and research experience in speech and language therapy in Ireland. She has used qualitative methodologies to explore a range of research interest such as the lived experience of communication disability, parental perspectives, identity construction, the voice of children with developmental speech and language disorders, and the social models of disability.

Francisco Javier Saavedra-Macías is currently Associate Professor in the Department of Experimental Psychology at the University of Seville, Spain, and a member of the Laboratory of Human Activity Research Group. He holds a PhD in psychology. He is also research fellow in the Andalusian Public Foundation for the Social Integration of Persons with Schizophrenia. His recent research is centred on the study caring processes in sociocultural settings, especially the discursive and communicational aspects.

Andrés Santamaría is Associate Professor in the Department of Experimental Psychology at the University of Seville, Spain, and a member of the research group Laboratory of Human Activity. He has a PhD in psychology. His recent research has centred on the cultural construction of autobiographical memory, cultural gender construction, and self-identity and migration.

Helena Taubner is a postdoctoral researcher at Halmstad University, Sweden, and has a PhD in health and lifestyle with a specialization in disability research. Her research interests include linguistic disabilities (aphasia), narrative agency, literacy practices, and identity.

Cecilie M.S. Thøgersen is a PhD student at Aalborg University and Neurocenter Østerskoven, Denmark, who specializes in the implementing of rehabilitation psychology in clinical practice. Her work has centred on how rehabilitation psychology can be implemented as a part of holistic rehabilitation after brain injury. Not only in relation to the person affected by the injury, but also the caregivers and relatives.

Åsa Wengelin is a professor of Swedish language at the University of Gothenburg, Sweden, and has a PhD in linguistics. Her research interests include reading and writing processes and practices, literacy acquisition and language disorders, with a special focus on written language and linguistic accessibility.

Sara Yuste holds a MA in neuropsychology at the University of Seville, and specializes in the intervention and therapy of people suffering. She is currently working as a neuropsychologist at the Association for the Rehabilitation of People with Aphasia (ARPA).

1 Narrative inquiry in disability research

Chalotte Glintborg and Manuel L. de la Mata

What is a narrative? There is no simple answer to this question. The term narrative refers broadly to a variety of traditions and scientific disciplines. Most often the term "narrative" is synonymous with "story". However, there are different definitions of what a narrative is and must contain to be a narrative, as we shall see in the following definitions.

A minimum definition of a narrative is that a narrative is a description of a chain of events put in the order they occur with the intention to make a point (Labov & Waletsky, 1967).

The narrative turn in social science

When reading about narrative inquiry, the *narrative turn* in social sciences is often mentioned. By "turn" is meant a change in direction from one way of thinking or being towards another.

The narrative turn in social sciences began in the early 1980s and encompassed a general anti-positivist and often humanist approach to the study of human psychology and culture (Plummer, 2001; Bruner, 1991; Riessman, 2008). In social sciences and psychology, the metaphoric approach to narrative, and the understanding of "life as narrative", were influential in the early days of the narrative turn. From this perspective, thus, human life can be conceived as a story. Like all stories, lives have plots. These plots (always "under construction") organize the facts of the past, make sense of the present, and project into the future.

One of the most outstanding representatives of the narrative turn in psychology is Jerome S. Bruner. Bruner was a central figure in the so-called "cognitive revolution" in the 1950s (see, for instance, Bruner, Goodnow, & Austin, 1956). Two decades later, in the 1980s, Bruner became very critical with cognitive psychology and its predominant (if not exclusive) interest in paradigmatic thinking (Bruner, 1986). Instead, he became interested in narrative thinking, since paradigmatic (logical) thinking is only part of human thinking. For Bruner, from birth, human beings make sense of the world of ourselves and other people by telling stories. Stories have characters, i.e. humanized characters, with motivations, mental states, goals, etc. We interpret other people's behaviour not in terms of cultural or stimulus–response relations, but in terms of mental states (beliefs, memories, expectations ...). If we analyse any trivial everyday conversation, we can only understand it by assuming that interlocutors are constantly attributing mental states to each other (intentionality).

For Bruner, narratives are also constituents of the self ("*self-making narrative*"), they are the raw material of life (Bruner, 2003b). From this perspective, we can find self and identity elements in any conversation, however trivial it may be. Stories are, thus, the core of human experience.

Since the 1980s, an increasing number of theorists in psychology and human sciences have embraced this narrative stance. Across the diversity of perspectives in this field, we can identify two general approaches (both theoretical and methodological) to narrative: small stories and big stories. Big stories are derived from interviews, clinical encounters, autobiographical writing, and other situations in which the individual is stimulated to reflect about her life from a somewhat distant perspective. Small stories, in contrast, derive from everyday social exchanges (Freeman, 2006). In general terms, the big stories approach is represented by theorists from psychology (personality, clinical psychology, and sometimes from cultural psychology) (Bruner, 2003a; Freeman, 2006; McAdams, 2001, 2015, among others). The small stories perspective, in turn, is represented by scholars from discursive psychology, sociolinguistics, etc. (Bamberg, 2004, 2011; Bamberg & Georgakopoulou, 2008; de Fina, Schiffrin, & Bamberg, 2006; de Fina & Georgakopoulou, 2012).

Among the representatives of the big stories approach we can mention Dan P. McAdams. His theory is based on the concept of "narrative identity". McAdams describes narrative identity as an internalized and evolving life story that people create about themselves – their own personal myths. When we intend people to understand us, we share our story, or parts of it, with them; when we want to know who another person is, we ask them to share part of their story. An individual's life story is not an exhaustive history of everything that has happened. Rather, we make what McAdams calls "narrative choices". Our stories tend to focus on the most extraordinary events, good and bad, because those are the experiences we need to make sense of and that shape us. But our interpretations may differ from person to person.

With regard to big stories, Freeman (2006) argues that big stories involve a sort of distancing from everyday life activities ("*life on holiday*"), a reflection about an individual's life. For that reason, they can be considered valuable tools for both individual reflection and narrative inquiry.

In contrast with the big stories approach, the "small stories movement" is grounded in a functional perspective on narrative and language use in general (Bamberg, 2011). Small stories researchers are interested in the social functions that narratives perform in the lives of people; in how people actually use stories in everyday, mundane situations in order to create (and perpetuate) a sense of who they are.

> Narratives are thus focused upon not as tools for reflecting on (chunks of) lives but as constructive means that are functional in the creation of

> characters in space and time, which in turn are instrumental for the creation of positions vis-à-vis co-conversationalists. Narratives are also aspects of situated language use, employed by speakers/narrators to position a display of contextualized identities.
>
> (Bamberg & Georgakopoulou, 2008, p. 379)

Small stories research, thus, is focused (and this is one of its most valuable contributions in this area) on the analysis of identity in practice, on how people display and rhetorically use identities in everyday discursive encounters. In other words, on the micro-genesis of identities in cultural practices/contexts. This approach contrasts with big story research, which analyses the stories as representations of world and identities within them (Bamberg, 2011, p. 16).

From our perspective these two approaches to identity are complementary and both are represented in this book. While big stories are often criticized for being "abstract" and artificial, we agree with Freeman (2006), who argues that, instead of being a problem, such "detached" nature of big stories creates opportunities for understanding and making sense of one's life beyond the vicissitudes/immediacy of the present.

Why use narrative inquiry in disability research?

Health and illness research is an area where narrative work is increasing. One example is the popular currency of "illness narratives" that has become part of the way we can relate to our own and other's illnesses. They can also include relatives' narratives on their illnesses and the effect on their lives. In the twenty-first century, different media platforms (i.e. websites, blogs, twitter, Facebook groups, etc.) has become a powerful means of spreading information, sharing emotions, and creating illness communities (Squire, Esin, & Burman, 2013). The medical-sociologist Arthur Frank suggested that our interest in illness narratives had to do with the needs of ill people to have their sufferings recognized. Personal illness narratives capture the individual's suffering in everyday situations in contrast to medical narratives. During the 1980s psychologists and sociologists explored the biographical disruptions and reconstitutions that follow serious long-term illness (Bury, 2001). All types of illnesses affect a person's experience of self and continuity, i.e. an acquired brain injury is not only a cognitive problem, but the person also changes his or her sense of self after this experience. Thus, illness is often experienced as an intruding event upon an ongoing life process. In narrative terms, the basic narrative threads of a person's life become broken and need to be reconstructed in telling new stories and revising previous stories. In such new storylines, it becomes possible to encompass both the illness and surrounding life events. Mattingly (2000) also describes how story-making and narratives are influential factors in reconstructing identity after illness. According to Mattingly, to tell a story about your illness can have a healing effect (Mattingly, 2000).

Narratives are one of the most important ways to make sense of our experiences. When ill, narratives offer an experiential space to weave together personal and medical concerns, where an individual can bind them together and integrate them in her life stories to figure out what their illness means for them and what can be done about it. Without the capacity to narrate, this process becomes difficult. The impact of communication disability on self-identity has received considerable attention in research investigating adjustment to aphasia (Shadden, 2005; Shadden & Koski, 2007; Silverman, 2011). Renegotiation of identity in circumstances of aphasia depends on how people with aphasia and their close relatives adapt to communication difficulties and, in this process, narratives can play an important role (Shadden, 2005).

However, there is an implicit assumption that individuals with neurological disabilities might find it hard to remember or narrate their past and may be unable to define a sense of self or be agentic. However, focusing on the person with the disorder as a participant engaged in interactions helps us conceptualize the consequences of the neurological disorder less as an individual problem but rather as something that is dealt with in everyday interactions together with other persons (Hyden, 2014). New trends in narrative inquiry includes studies on narrative identity in individuals with Alzheimer's Dementia (AD). Much research in AD, and other neurological diseases, has focused on describing and explaining the declining cognitive and linguistic abilities. Little research has focused on the ways persons with AD cope with these losses. To add a narrative approach to AD helps us to conceptualize the consequences of AD less as an individual problem than as something that is dealt with in everyday interactions together with other persons. In a unique study, Kemper and colleagues (1995) found that:

> patients with AD are able to communicate more effectively with their spouses' help and assistance than they are able to alone. Spouses can provide contextual cues for the participants, settings, and significant events in the lives of the patient with AD.
>
> (Kemper, Lyons, & Anagnopoulos, 1995, p. 219)

These findings are in line with sociocultural traditions, for instance Vygotsky, who argued that the interaction between persons is the base for the child's (and adult's) cognitive, linguistic, and social development (Bruner, 1985; Lave and Wenger, 1991). Narrative inquiry has also been used to explore children's experiences. For example, it has been used to explore children's experiences of school (Westling Allodi, 2002), reading (Davis, 2007), bullying (Bosacki, Marini, & Dane, 2006), sexual abuse (Mossige, Jensen, Gulbrandsen, Reichelt, & Tjersland, 2005) and identity construction and meaning-making in children with speech and language disorders (Lyons & Roulstone, 2017). A narrative approach allows for a rich description of experiences and an exploration of the meanings that the participants derive from their experiences. Narrative inquiry amplifies voices that may have otherwise remained silent. Thus, the aim of this book is to utilize storytelling as a way of communicating the participants' realities to a larger and more in-depth understanding of the particulars of the participants' points of view. The knowledge gained can offer the reader a deeper understanding of the subject material and extra insight to apply the stories to their own context. Narrative inquiry has an underlying philosophy that enables the illumination of real people in real settings through the "painting" of their stories.

References

Bamberg, M. (2004). Talk, small stories, and adolescent identities. *Human Development*, 47, 366–369.

Bamberg, M. (2011). Who am I: Narration and its contribution to identity. *Theory & Psychology*, 21, 3–24. doi:10.1177/0959354309355852.

Bamberg, M. & Georgakopoulou, A. (2008). Small stories as a new perspective in narrative and identity analysis. *Text & Talk*, 3, 377–396.

Bosacki, S., Marini, Z., & Dane, A. (2006). Voices from the classroom: Pictorial and narrative representations of children's bullying experiences. *Journal of Moral Education*, 35(2), 231–245.

Bruner, J. (1985). *Child's talk: Learning to use language*. New York: W.W. Norton & Co.

Bruner, J. (1986). *Actual minds, possible worlds*. Cambridge, MA: Harvard University Press.

Bruner, J. (1991). The narrative construction of reality. *Critical Inquiry*, 18, 1–21.

Bruner, J.S. (2003a). *Making stories: Life, literature, law*. Cambridge, MA: Harvard University Press.

Bruner, J.S. (2003b). Self-making narratives. In R. Fivush & C.A. Haden (Eds.), *Autobiographical memory and the construction of a narrative self: Developmental and cultural perspectives* (pp. 209–225). Mahwah: Lawrence Erlbaum Associates.

Bruner, J.S., Goodnow, J.J., & Austin, G.A. (1956). *A study of thinking*. New York: Wiley.

Bury, M. (2001). Illness narratives: Facts or fiction. *Sociology of Health and Illness*, 23, 263–285.

Davis, P. (2007). Storytelling as a democratic approach to data collection: Interviewing children about reading. *Educational Research*, 49(2), 169–184.

De Fina, A. & Georgakopoulou, A. (2015). Introduction. In A. de Fina & A. Georgakopoulou (Eds.), *Handbook of narrative analysis* (pp. 1–17). New York: Wiley.

De Fina, A., Schiffrin, D., & Bamberg, M. (Eds.) (2006). *Discourse and identity*. Cambridge: Cambridge University Press.

Freeman, M. (2006). Life on "holiday"? In defense of big stories. *Narrative Inquiry*, 16, 131–138.

Hyden, L.C. (2014). How to do things with others: Joint activities involving persons with Alzheimer's disease. In L.C. Hyden, H. Lindeman, & J. Brockmeir (Eds.), *Beyond loss: Dementia, identity, personhood* (pp. 137–154). New York: Oxford University Press.

Kemper, S., Lyons, K., & Anagnopoulos, C. (1995). Joint storytelling by patients with Alzheimer's disease and their spouses. *Discourse Process*, 20, 205–217.

Labov, W. & Waletzky, J. (1967). Narrative analysis. In J. Helm (Ed.), *Essays on the verbal and visual arts* (pp. 12–44). Seattle: University of Washington Press. Reprinted in the *Journal of Narrative and Life History*, 7, 3–38(1997).

Lave, J. & Wenger, E. (1991). *Situated learning: Legitimate peripheral participation.* New York: Cambridge University Press.

Lyons, R. & Roulstone, S. (2017). Labels, identity and narratives in children with primary speech and language impairments. *International Journal of Speech-Language Pathology*, 5, 503–518.

McAdams, D.P. (2001). The psychology of life stories. *Review of General Psychology*, 5 (2), 100–122.

McAdams, D.P. (2015). Three lines of personality development: A conceptual itinerary. *European Psychologist*, 20, 252–264.

Mattingly, C. (2000). Emergent narratives. In C. Mattingly & L. Garro (Eds.), *Narrative and the cultural construction of illness and healing* (pp. 181–211). Berkeley: University of California Press.

Mossige, S., Jensen, T., Gulbrandsen, W., Reichelt, S., & Burman, C. (2005). Children's narratives of sexual abuse: What characterises them and how do they contribute to meaning-making? *Narrative Inquiry*, 15(2), 377–404.

Plummer, K. (2001). *Documents of life 2: An invitation to a critical humanism.* London: Sage.

Riessman, C.K. (2008). *Narrative methods for the human sciences.* Newbury Park: Sage.

Shadden, B.B. (2005). Aphasia as identity theft: Theory and practice. *Aphasiology*, 19, 211–223.

Shadden, B.B. & Kosky, P.R. (2007). Social construction of self for persons with aphasia: When language as a cultural tool is impaired. *Journal of Medical Speech-Language Pathology*, 15, 99–105.

Silverman, M. (2011). The dignity of struggle. *Topics in Stroke Rehabilitation*, 18, 134–138.

Squire, C., Esin, C., & Burman, C. (2013). "You are here": Visual autobiographies, cultural-spatial positioning, and resources for urban living. *Sociological Research Online*, 18(3), 1.

Westling Allodi, M. (2002). Children's experiences of school: Narratives of Swedish children with and without learning difficulties. *Scandinavian Journal of Educational Research*, 46(2), 181–205.

2 Narrative identity is social context

Manuel L. de la Mata, Andrés Santamaría, Mercedes Cubero and Rosario Cubero

Before exploring the use of narratives in relation to different forms of disability, this chapter presents our conception of identity-self. This conception is, in general terms, coincident with the notions of identity adopted in the chapters of this book. Before describing in detail this conception, we will start with a brief chronological-conceptual journey through the notion of identity-self in psychology and social sciences. Far from being a comprehensive review of the evolution of the concepts, we will try to identify some important traditions and theoretical approaches. Among them, we will especially focus on narrative approaches to identity-self.

After that short journey through the concepts of self and identity we will develop in more detail our conception of identity-self as distributed (situated), narrative, and dialogical. This conception is based on scholars and theories such as McAdams, Bruner, rhetorical approaches to identity, and the Dialogical Self Theory.

After presenting the conceptual basis of our conception we are going to address two issues that are, in our view, critical for any theorization about narrative self-identity: the tension between continuity versus change and between consistency and situatedness in self-identity and the role of the microsocial versus the macrosocial.

Introduction: the notion of identity-self in psychology: a controversial concept

The notions of identity and self have a long and controversial history in psychology and social sciences. As complex and heterogeneous concepts, they have been addressed by different disciplines and from different theoretical perspectives. Although this is not the place for a comprehensive review of the evolution of the concepts, we need to briefly refer to some of the main theoretical traditions in this study. While in some cases the authors have predominantly use the term self, in others they have employed the term identity (or identities, in plural).

The first author to speak about the self in psychology was William James (1890). James' notion of self was based on the distinction between the *I* (the self as "knower" or the self as subject) and the *me* (the object to be known) (Hermans & Gieser, 2011). After William James, the interest for the self in mainstream psychology decayed and even the use of the term practically disappeared during the first half of the twentieth century. However, it persisted in sociology, within the theoretical approach of symbolic interactionism, in the works of George Herbert Mead (1934). Mead maintained the distinction between the I and the me, although he introduced some changes with regard to James' theory. In this vein, Mead rejected a vision of the self as a mere reproducer of social convention, highlighting its capacity for cultural innovation (assigned to the I). The *me*, in contrast, was to be defined by the rules and conventions of the "generalized other". By introducing this concept, Mead was emphasizing the intrinsically social nature of the self. For Mead (and for William James, as well), the self could not be conceived as an isolated entity, since the core of the self includes the others, both the close others and society and its institutions.

It was during the beginning of the second half of the twentieth century that the emergence of the so-called dramaturgic movement and, in particular ethnomethodology, with Ervin Goffman (1967) as its main representative, put the self at the centre of the stage, again. In coincidence with Mead, ethnomethodology gave the priority to the social self. We must note that the conception of individual and culture in ethnomethodology is based in the dramaturgic metaphor: people are actors in a play that is represented before different audiences. The existence of these different audiences and scenarios lead individuals to adopt (perform) different identities. This implies to consider the self more as a consequence than a cause of the performance. From this perspective, thus, there is not an enduring sense of the self (Swann & Bosson, 2010).

During the 1970s and, especially, the 1980s, a neo-Jamesian conception of the self emerged in psychology (Swann & Bosson, 2010). This conception has recovered some of the central elements of James' notion of the self, including the recognition of its enduring dimension. After this theoretical turn, the study of identity-self has consolidated in social and personality psychology.

In other areas of psychology, the term identity, more than self, has been predominant. An example of this is the tradition rooted in Erik Erikson (1950, 1968), and the tradition of the study of social identities, based on the social identity theory proposed by Tajfel and Turner (1986) and the self-categorization theory represented by Turner (1987; 1989, cited in Ellemers, Spears, & Doosje, 2002). This tradition is focused on the role of social identities in intergroup relations (Vignoles et al., 2012).

Within the tradition of study of the self in social and personality psychology, we can make a distinction between cognitive and narrative approaches. Cognitive approaches conceive the self in terms of mental representations (Baumeister, 1998; Swann & Bosson, 2010), namely, as a set of cognitive structures (both explicit or implicit) that enable the individual to make sense of the world s/he lives in. These ideas and beliefs about what one is and may become constitute self-concept (Oyserman, Elmore, & Smith, 2012). Together with the dimension of self-knowledge, the self also includes a social component (social being and reputation) and a self-regulation dimension (Baumeister, 1998).

Within the narrative approaches, we must mention authors such as Dan P. McAdams, Katherine Nelson, Robyn Fivush, and Jerome S. Bruner, among many others. McAdams has proposed a multilevel approach to personality in which identity represents the third/highest level of analysis. In this vein, McAdams distinguishes between self and identity and defines identity as a life story (McAdams, 1993, 2001). McAdams' approach, influenced by Erikson, as well, has put the emphasis on the role of cultural factors (and, specifically, cultural narratives) on identity (McAdams, 2006; McAdams & McLean, 2013; McLean & Syed, 2015).

The focus on the role of culture is characteristic of authors such as Katherine Nelson and Robyn Fivush, from developmental psychology (Nelson & Fivush, 2004; Fivush & Nelson, 2006; Fivush, 2011), as well. While it is possible to trace back Erikson's influences in these authors, their main interest is to develop a sociocultural theory of the self, strongly influenced by the works of Lev S. Vygotsky (1978; Wertsch, 1985).

The interest for the cultural dimension of the self is shared with authors and theories from cross-cultural psychology, anthropology, and cultural psychology. Cross-cultural approaches to the self are largely influenced by the seminal work of Markus and Kitayama (1991) and their distinction between the independent and interdependent self, subsequently developed and criticized by scholars such as Kagitçibaşi (2007, 2017), Keller (2007), and Greenfield (2009), among others. Together with the theories developed in cross-cultural psychology, we can also mention some approaches from anthropology (Shweder & Bourne, 1984). Finally, within the field of cultural psychology, we cannot forget the contribution of Jerome S. Bruner (1990, 2002, 2003). In the next section we are going to further develop Bruner's conception of the self.

Within narrative approaches to identity-self, there are also another two lines that have contributed to theorizing about identity-self and are represented in this book. We can call them rhetorical and dialogical approaches. Although both share a large number of ideas with the narrative approaches mentioned so far, it is interesting to highlight some specific contributions from each line.

The antecedents of rhetorical approaches to identity-self can be traced back to theories such as Wittgenstein's philosophy of language, post-modern philosophy or post-structuralist social theory (Vignoles, Schwartz & Luyckx, 2012) and discursive psychology (Potter & Wetherell, 1987; Edwards & Potter, 1992; Wetherell, 2010; Nentwich & Morison, 2018), among others. Social positioning theory, which represents a major contribution to the study of narrative identity, can be framed in this perspective (see Bamberg, 1997, 2011 or de Fina and Georgakopoulou, 2015 for a more extensive account of this theory).

Finally, dialogical approaches to narrative self are represented by Dialogical Self Theory (Hermans, Rijks, & Kempen, 1993; Hermans, 2001; Hermans & Gieser, 2011). This neo-Bakhtinian (Bakhtin, 1986) approach considers the self as a dynamic multiplicity of I-positions that enter into dialogue. As we shall develop later, these I-positions that constitute the self are legitimized by individual and social voices, so that the self is constituted as a true "society of mind".

Although the above distinction among traditions and theoretical approaches is useful for the purpose of organizing a complex and heterogeneous field like this, we must not forget the considerable overlap among the previous lines, which have extensively influenced each other. This intersection makes it in many cases difficult to frame specific theories and authors within one line or another.

Besides the conceptual roots of the theories, an important issue that characterizes and differentiates them is the position they take in relation to the dilemmas between stability and change and adjustment to situations (situatedness) of identity-self. In this regard, while cognitive theories emphasize the stability of the self through time and situations (taking what Swann and Bossom have called a neo-Jamesian approach), in general, narrative approaches hold a different position towards this dilemma, putting the emphasis on situatedness (Bamberg, 2011; de Fina & Georgakopoulou, 2015) and/or defining stability in terms of narrative continuity or coherence (Habermas & Bluck, 2000; McAdams & McLean, 2013). In the next section we shall return to this issue.

A distributed, narrative, and dialogical view of self-identity

The main antecedents of our notion of the self can be found in James and Mead, as well as Bakhtin. From this perspective, rather than considering the self as a cognitive entity (a set of knowledge representations, Baumeister, 1998), something homogeneous and stable located in the individual, we conceive the self as a dynamic construction, with three main characteristics: situated (distributed), narrative, and dialogical. In the following we are going to refer to each of these characteristics

With regard to the situated character of self-identity, Bruner (1995) advocates for the distributed nature of the self. For him, the self can be defined as a "sum and swarm of participations" (1990, p. 107). For Bruner, the self is continuously reconstructed to adjust to the characteristics and needs of the situations in which human beings participate (Bruner, 2002).

As Bruner (1995) claims:

> there is no such thing as an intuitively obvious and essential self … Rather we constantly construct and reconstruct ourselves to meet the needs of situations we encounter, and we do so with the guidance of our memories of the past and our hopes and fears for the future. Telling oneself about oneself is like making up a story about who and what we are, what has happened, and why we are doing what we are doing.
>
> (p. 210)

Bruner's emphasis on the distributed nature of the self has points in common with small theories approaches to narrative identity (Bamberg, 2006; Georgakopoulou, 2006; Bamberg & Georgakopoulou, 2008; de Fina & Georgakopoulou, 2015, see Chapter 1 in this volume). This approach puts the focus on the study of "narratives-in-interaction, the way stories surface in everyday conversation (small stories), as the locus where identities are continuously practiced and tested out" (Bamberg, 2011, p. 15). These stories are situated to meet the requirements of the context and the purposes they are told for.

The above idea connects with the second quality of the self, its narrative structure, what Bruner calls the "storied self". For Bruner (1990), when we ask people how they are, they usually tell a variety of stories, using the traditional elements of narrative, conceived both as a way of discourse and as a way of organizing experience (a way of thinking). These narratives involve a sequence of actions carried out by characters who act on behalf of mental states (beliefs, emotions, memories, intentions, expectations ...). In this sense, for Bruner every story includes two complementary aspects or dimensions (two landscapes, in Bruner's words), the landscape of action (including goals, causes and temporal sequence) and the landscape of consciousness (that includes motives, mental states, motivations and evaluations).

In a related vein, McAdams (2001; McAdams & Olson, 2010), distinguishes self and identity. While for McAdams the notion of self is broader and comprises not only narrative components (i.e. self-concept, self-esteem, etc.), identity is a life story. In McAdams' words:

> identity itself takes the form of a story, complete with setting, scenes, character, plot, and theme. In late adolescence and young adulthood, people living in modern societies begin to reconstruct the personal past, perceive the present, and anticipate the future in terms of an internalised and evolving self-story, an integrative narrative of self that provides modern life with some modicum of psychosocial unity and purpose.
>
> (McAdams, 2001, p. 101)

As we shall develop in the next pages, narrative provides a solution to the dilemmas of continuity versus change and consistency versus situatedness. Instead of attributing any kind of pre-existing continuity or consistency to the self, narrative approaches conceive continuity and consistency as narrative constructions. In this sense, rhetorical approaches state that when confronted with the criticism of lack of continuity or consistency between situations, people construct accounts (stories) to "demonstrate" consistency or, at least, to make the changes undergone across time and situations understandable (see, for instance, Billig, 1987 or Edwards and Potter, 1992 for a further elaboration of this issue).

Narratives of the self are socially, culturally, and historically framed. In their exchanges with significant others in sociocultural settings, individuals appropriate cultural narratives from the "menu of stories" (McAdams, 2006) provided by culture. These master narratives provide the guidelines for the development of narrative identity (McAdams & McLean, 2013; McLean & Syed, 2015).

The third characteristic of the self mentioned above is its dialogical nature. This idea has its roots in the works of the Russian semiologist Mikhail Bakhtin (Bakhtin, 1973, 1986). For Bakhtin, language is, by definition, polyphonic. Any linguistic production (utterance), although produced by a specific individual, expresses a set of voices (besides the individual's). These "speaking personalities" or "speaking consciousness" (Emerson & Holquist, 1981, in Wertsch, 1991) involve viewpoints, worldviews that individuals assume and express through their own voices.

Based on Bakhtin's ideas, Hermans has proposed the notion of dialogical self. For the Dialogical Self Theory (Hermans, 2001, 2003; Hermans & Gieser, 2011), the self can be understood as a "*dynamic multiplicity of I-positions*" (Hermans & Gieser, 2011, p. 2) that individuals adopt in relation to and involving the significant others. But when people speak they do not only position themselves in relation to other people. They also position other people, which, in turn, do the same with them. The notion of position is then, very dynamic, intrinsically linked to acting in specific contexts and changing with time.

From this perspective, the I emerges from its encounters with others within the social and cultural context. In these encounters the I is moving from one position to another, depending on the characteristics and requirements of the situations. Moreover, I-positions are *voiced* (in Bakhtin's terms), which means that movements and exchanges between I-positions imply dialogical exchanges between voices. For Hermans and Gieser, the voices behave like the interacting characters in a story or a movie, involved in complex processes of agreement–disagreement, negotiations, conflicts, etc.

The vision of the self presented above requires, in our opinion, a multilevel approach to its analysis. From our perspective, the study of the self cannot be exclusively focused on the analysis of the individual, as if it were a separate entity, regardless of the interactions with other people and the sociocultural practices people participate in. On the contrary, we assume that the very definition of the self and, therefore, its study, must be carried out at three planes of analysis: the individual, the interpersonal, and the sociocultural plane. This theoretical-methodological approach is at the core of the sociocultural approach to the human mind (Vygotsky, 1978; Wertsch, 1985, 1991). According to this theoretical framework, the definition and the study of self-identity must go beyond the isolated individual and encompasses the individual, interpersonal, and sociocultural levels. In other words, the analysis of the identity processes demands a vision of the self that is not exhausted in the study of the resources, strategies, and capacities of individuals. It must integrate both the analysis of the relationships that people maintain with their close environment (which can act as models and as referents for identity processes), as well as that of the cultural discourses and ideologies in which the narratives of the self are framed. To construct the narratives of the self, individuals appropriate cultural discourses and ideologies, whether to identify with or to resist them.

Key questions in the study of self-identity

After presenting the conceptual basis of our conception we need to address some important issues in the study of narrative self-identity. These issues are more or less explicitly dealt with across the chapters of this book. We refer to the tension between continuity versus change and between consistency and situatedness in self-identity and to the role of the microsocial versus the macrosocial in self-identity.

From our perspective, the tension between continuity versus change is at the core of identity construction and development and, for that reason, needs to be addressed in identity theorization. For Bamberg (2011), the first dilemma that any claim of identity must address concerns a sense of sameness across time in the face of constant change through life. Since the theme of this book is identity and disability, the next chapters describe situations in which people face experiences that represent a rupture both in their lives and of those who live with them. For that reason, the dilemma of continuity versus change or rupture, always at the core of identity development, acquires, in these cases, a paramount importance. In this regard, while cognitive theories about the self emphasize continuity (in the line of what Swann & Bosson (2010) have called a neo-Jamesian approach to the self), narrative approaches put the focus on change and adjustment to situations and/or re-conceptualize continuity in narrative terms (as narrative coherence, for example). For Bruner (1990), narratives enable people to make sense of the breaches with the canonical. Given that suffering a brain stroke, being diagnosed with AD or aphasia or the rise of any other type of disability, undoubtedly represent a break in individuals and families' lives, developing a story of the self (which, by definition, includes the others) that makes sense of this breach and integrates both continuity and change in life becomes a necessity in these cases. From a theoretical-methodological perspective, narrative approaches to identity become especially appropriate to account for the way individuals and families face the challenge for identity associated with disability. Let's briefly refer to these approaches more specifically.

As we explained above, McAdams (2001) conceptualizes identity as a life story. Once individuals in Western societies construct a life story after adolescence, these life stories are continuously being re-created through the life course. Notwithstanding this continuous change, when faced with the question: "Am I the same person that I was ten/twenty years ago?" people need to give a positive answer or, alternatively, be able to trace back the changes since now to the past. This "journey back" from the present to the past is made possible by autobiographical memory (Nelson, 2003; Santamaría & Montoya, 2008). To achieve the goal of construing continuity, life stories have to be coherent. The concept of narrative coherence goes beyond coherence between sentences, and refers to the relationships between the elements of a text (the life story, in this case) at a moment in time. According to Habermas (Habermas & Bluck, 2000; Habermas & de Silveira, 2008), coherence should not be confounded with stability over time. For this author, life stories must comply with four types of coherence: temporal, causal, thematic, and coherence with the cultural concept of biography.

In rhetorical approaches to narrative identity, continuity and consistency are conceptualized in a different way. For these approaches, the focus is to study what participants do with narratives (de Fina & Georgakopoulou, 2015), that is to go beyond the analysis of narratives as texts to analyse the social practice of narration in sociocultural contexts (Bamberg, 2011). Since narratives are accounts constructed in specific contexts that serve specific rhetorical purposes, the task of narrative analysis is, rather than identifying the elements that remain stable across different versions of "the same story", to establish how narrative accounts are linked to the characteristics of the specific situations (the participants, the goals, the social practices in which the situation is embedded ...) and the ongoing actions in which these narrations are performed (Billig, 1987; Edwards, 1997; Wiggins & Potter, 2008; Bamberg, 2011). From this standpoint, consistency is regarded as a rhetorical issue. When questioned about the eventual existence of inconsistences in different narrative accounts of events, people justify these inconsistencies by using a variety of rhetorical resources (denying the contradictions, claiming that the changes are forced by the situations, etc.).

Dialogical Self Theory also emphasizes the situated character of identities. In this sense, since I-positions are related to specific situations and practices that individuals participate in, this notion acknowledges the multiplicity of the self (Hermans & Gieser, 2011). Notwithstanding that, Dialogical Self theorists claim that the consistency and unity of the self is preserved, as well. To reconcile both aspects, the theory speaks of the existence of both decentring and centring movements of the I-positions. The decentring movements of the I involve taking new positions across time and space. These new I-positions would have relative autonomy, their own specific history in the self, and would show different developmental pathways. In a complementary way, the I appropriates some of these positions while rejecting others (centring movements).

At the same time, to account for the way that the self integrates different and sometimes conflicting I-positions, Dialogical Self Theory proposes three notions: third position, meta-position and promoter position. A third position let the self reconcile (eliminate, reduce, or mitigate) the conflict between two contradictory positions. A meta-position, in turn, requires a reflective exercise by which the individual take some distance from one or several positions. This also enables the subject to look at different positions, making their linkages visible. Adopting a meta-position may also help to solve eventual conflicts between I-positions, facilitating the further development of the self.

Finally, the concept of promoter position can be considered equivalent to meta-position with regard to a temporal perspective. Typically, significant others (whether close or distant, real or imagined) may play the role of promoter positions, exerting long-lasting influences as promoters or anti-promoters, thereby facilitating the development of existing positions or generating new ones (Hermans & Gieser, 2011). By doing so, promoter positions have important influence on the development of the self.

Another key issue is related to the role of sociocultural influences on identity-self. In this sense, while all narrative approaches to identity-self attach special importance to social and cultural factors, some interesting nuances appear when we compare the way they consider this issue.

Authors such as McAdams (and Bruner, as well) are mostly interested in the role of macrosocial (cultural) influences in narrative identity-self. In this vein, McAdams has focused on analysing individuals' life stories to identify specific plots from the menu of stories provided by culture. Among these plots, McAdams refers to the "redemptive self" (McAdams, 2006) as characteristic of American culture.

The redemptive self is an example of *master narrative* (McLean & Syed, 2015). For McLean and Syed, the notion of a master narrative allows the researcher to locate the study of identity in culture. For McLean and Syed, master narratives are "culturally shared stories that guide thoughts, beliefs, values, and behaviours" (McLean & Syed, 2015, p. 323). They are not personal narratives, but broader culture-specific stories that individuals can internalize or resist, whether consciously or unconsciously. Master narratives are characterized by five general principles (ubiquity, utility, invisibility, rigidity, and compulsory nature).

Rhetorical traditions, in turn, highlight the situated character of narrative identities. They pay special attention to the immediate context (here-and-now) in the process of production of narrative identity (de Fina & Georgakopoulou, 2015). In this sense, Bamberg (2004) has proposed three levels of positioning analysis. At level 1 he proposes to scrutinize the linguistic means used to establish the characters and their relations within the story. In Bamberg's words, this aims to answer the question "How are the characters depicted, and what is the story about (its theme)?" (p. 336). This corresponds to the consideration of "narrative as text" (Georgakopoulou, 2006). In the second level (positioning level 2), the focus is the analysis of the interactive work between the participants in the interaction in which narration is produced. For Bamberg, the relevant question for this level would be why a particular story is being told at a specific point in the interaction. In so doing, the interviewee is positioning herself in front of the interviewer.

Finally, positioning level 3 involves transcending both the narrative text and the situation of narration to answer the question "Who am I?" (Bamberg, 2004, p. 336). In other words, the narrator positions herself vis-à-vis cultural discourses (by embracing, criticizing, resisting them). In sum, performing an identity in sociocultural context.

The Dialogical Self Theory (Hermans & Gieser, 2011) addresses the issue through the notions of I-positions and voices. By looking at the movements from one position to another over time, Dialogical Self scholars can examine how identities are performed at the microsocial (face-to-face) level. On the other hand, identifying the voices that articulate the I-positions (Santamaría, Cubero, Prados, & de la Mata, 2013) allow researchers to analyse how cultural narratives resonate in individuals' narratives, enabling them to frame the identities performed in everyday real situations in the cultural context.

Conclusion

In this chapter we have presented a theoretical approach in which identity-self is conceptualized as distributed and situated, narrative and dialogical. From this perspective, identities-selves cannot be understood and, thereby, studied only at the individual level. Instead, we need to consider social interactions (including the interaction between interviewer and interviewee) and the cultural practices in which these interactions take place. Through participation in these socioculturally framed interactions, people engage in a continuous process of (re) constructing their life stories, vis-à-vis the social discourses (master narratives) that provide guidelines for these life stories. Far from being a simple internalisation of the dominant master narratives, this process involves very complex and bi-directional relations in which individuals embrace, resist, contest, and transform master narratives from the menu of stories of their culture (McAdams, 2006). Narrative approaches to identity-self provide, in our view, both theoretical and methodological tools to account for such processes. In the methodological plane, the methods and techniques employed are predominantly qualitative (semi-structured interview, focus-groups, observation of everyday interactions, conversation analysis). Our proposal of employing qualitative methodologies for the study of identity-self in relation to disability does not mean the rejection of quantitative methodologies. On the contrary, we think that quantitative and qualitative methodologies, rather than contradictory, are complementary, as they enable to analyse different dimensions of identities and to answer different questions about them. With regard to this issue, we agree with Monrad (2013) when she claims that both kinds of methods enable the study of different aspects of identity while remaining blind to others. More specifically, for this author quantitative survey-based methodologies that rely on self-report and closed-ended questions, such as questionnaires and scales, allow us to carry out systematic and standardized comparisons among individuals, making it possible to examine patterns of identification in large populations and groups. These methods, however, do not allow to examine the performative, embodied, and narrative character of identities (the processes of construction-negotiation of identities in sociocultural settings), but "a condensation of some thoughts and feelings with regard to the actual perception of self as performer of a specific role in the form of abstract adjectives" (Monrad, 2013, p. 350). Qualitative methodologies, in turn, have demonstrated their utility to account for the meaning that individuals (re)construct about themselves in sociocultural settings. This includes aspects such as the narrative construction of continuity–discontinuity in life stories, the way in which individuals appropriate master narratives (including how they resist them) to construct their narrative identities-selves and the way identities are performed in ongoing social interactions.

Acknowledgements

This chapter was written with the support of the research project funded by the Government of Spain [PSI2016–80112–P] entitled "Challenges of the self: Identity reconstruction in situations of inequality and social exclusion".

References

Bakhtin, M. (1973). *Problems of Dostoevsky's poetics.* Translated by R.W. Rotsel. Ann Arbor: Ardis.

Bakhtin, M. (1986). *Speech genres and other late essays.* Austin: University of Texas Press.

Bamberg, M. (1997). Positioning between structure and performance. *Journal of Narrative and Life History*, 7, 335–342.

Bamberg, M. (2004). Talk, small stories, and adolescent identities. *Human Development*, 47, 366–369.

Bamberg, M. (2006). Stories: Big or small? Why do we care? *Narrative Inquiry*, 16(1), 147–155. doi:10.1075/ni.16.1.18bam.

Bamberg, M. (2011). Who am I: Narration and its contribution to identity. *Theory & Psychology*, 21, 3–24. doi:10.1177/0959354309355852.

Bamberg, M. & Georgakopoulou, A. (2008). Small stories as a new perspective in narrative and identity analysis. *Text & Talk*, 3, 377–396.

Baumeister, R.F. (1998). The self. In D.Y.T. Gilbert, S.T. Fiske, & G. Lindzey (Eds.), *The handbook of social psychology*, Vol. 1 (4th Edition) (pp. 680–740). Boston: McGraw-Hill.

Billig, M. (1987). *Arguing and thinking: A rhetorical approach to social psychology.* Cambridge: Cambridge University Press.

Bruner, J. (1986). *Actual minds, possible worlds.* Cambridge, MA: Harvard University Press.

Bruner, J.S. (1990). *Acts of meaning*, Vol. 3. Cambridge, MA: Harvard University Press.

Bruner, J. (1995). Meaning and self in cultural perspective. In D. Bakhurst & C. Spinowich (Eds.), *The social self* (pp. 18–29). London: Sage Publications.

Bruner, J.S. (2002). *Making stories: Law, literature, life.* New York: Farrar, Straus and Giroux.

Bruner, J.S. (2003). Self-making narratives. In R. Fivush & C.A. Haden (Eds.), *Autobiographical memory and the construction of a narrative self: Developmental and cultural perspectives* (pp. 209–225) Mahwah: Lawrence Erlbaum Associates.

De Fina, A. & Georgakopoulou, A. (2015). Introduction. In A. de Fina & A. Georgakopoulou (Eds.), *Handbook of narrative analysis* (pp. 1–17). New York: Wiley.

Edwards, D. (1997). *Discourse and cognition*. London: Sage.

Edwards, D. & Potter, J. (1992). *Discursive psychology.* London: Sage.

Ellemers, N., Spears, R., & Doosje, B. (2002). Self and social identity. *Annual Review of Psychology*, 53, 161–186. doi:10.1146/annurev.psych.53.100901.135228.

Erikson, E.H. (1950). *Childhood in society.* New York: Norton.

Erikson, E.H. (1968). *Identity: Youth and crisis.* New York: Norton.

Fivush, R. (2011). The development of autobiographical memory. *Annual Review of Psychology*, 62, 559–582. http://dx.doi.10.1146/annurev.psych.121208.131702.

Fivush, R. & Nelson, K. (2006). Parent-child reminiscing locates the self in the past. *British Journal of Developmental Psychology*, 24, 235–251. http://dx.doi.org/10.1348/026151005X57747.

Georgakopoulou, A. (2006). Thinking big with small stories in narrative and identity analysis. *Narrative Inquiry*, 16(1), 122–130. https://doi.org/10.1075/ni.16.1.16geo.

Goffman, E. (1967). *Interaction ritual: Essays on face-to-face behavior.* Garden City: Doubleday.

Greenfield, P.M. (2009). Linking social change and developmental change: Shifting. pathways of human development. *Developmental Psychology*, 45, 401–418. http://doi.10.1037/a0014726.

Habermas, T. & Bluck, S. (2000). Getting a life: The development of the life story in adolescence. *Psychological Bulletin*, 126, 748–769.

Habermas, T. & de Silveira, C. (2008). The development of global coherence in life narratives across adolescence: Temporal, causal, and thematic aspects. *Developmental Psychology*, 44(3), 707–721. doi:10.1037/0012-1649.44.3.707.

Hermans, H.J. (2001). The dialogical self: Toward a theory of personal and cultural positioning. *Culture & Psychology*, 7(3), 243–281.

Hermans, H.J. (2003). The construction and reconstruction of a dialogical self. *Journal of Constructivist Psychology*, 16(2), 89–130. https://doi:10.1080/10720530390117902.

Hermans, H.J. & Gieser, T. (Eds.) (2011). *Handbook of dialogical self theory.* Cambridge: Cambridge University Press.

Hermans, H.J., Rijks, T.I., & Kempen, H.J. (1993). Imaginal dialogues in the self: Theory and method. *Journal of Personality*, 61(2), 207–236.

Kagitçibaşi, C. (2007). *Family, self and human development across cultures: Theory and applications.* Mahwah: Lawrence Erlbaum Associates.

Kagitçibaşi, C. (2017). Doing psychology with a cultural lens: A half-century journey. *Perspectives on Psychological Science*, 12(5), 824–832. https://doi.org/10.1177/17456916177009.

Keller, H. (2007). *Children development across cultures.* New York: Lawrence Erlbaum Associates.

James, W. (1890/1981). *The principles of psychology*, Vol 12. Cambridge, MA: Harvard University Press.

McAdams, D.P. (1993). *The stories we lived by: Personal myths and the making of the self.* New York: Guilford Press.

McAdams, D.P. (2001). The psychology of life stories. *Review of General Psychology*, 5, 100–122. doi:10.1037/1089–2680.5.2.100.

McAdams, D.P. (2006). *The redemptive self: Stories Americans live by.* New York: Oxford University Press.

McAdams, D.P. & McLean, K.C. (2013) Narrative identity. *Current Directions in Psychological Science*, 22(3), 233–238. doi:10.1177/0963721413475622.

McAdams, D.P. & Olson, B.D. (2010). Personality development: Continuity and change over the life course. *Annual Review of Psychology*, 61, 517–542. doi:10.1146/annurev.psych.093008.100507.

McLean, K.C. & Syed, M. (2015). Personal, master, and alternative narratives: An integrative framework for understanding identity development in context. *Human Development*, 58(6), 318–349. doi:10.1159/000445817.

Markus, H.R. & Kitayama, S. (1991). Culture and the self: Implications for cognition, emotion, and motivation. *Psychological Review*, 98, 224–253. doi:10.1037/0033–0295X.98.2.224.

Mead, G.H. (1934). *Mind, self and society*, Vol. 111. Chicago: University of Chicago Press.

Monrad, M. (2013). On a scale of one to five, who are you? Mixed methods in identity research. *Acta Sociologica*, 56, 347–360. doi:10.1177/0001699313481368.

Nelson, K. (2003). Narrative and self, myth and memory: Emergence of the cultural self. In R. Fivush & C.A. Haden (Eds.), *Autobiographical memory and the construction of a narrative self: Developmental and cultural perspectives* (pp. 3–28). Mahwah: Lawrence Erlbaum Associates.

Nelson, K. & Fivush, R. (2004). The emergence of autobiographical memory: A social cultural developmental theory. *Psychological Review*, 111(2), 486–511. https://doi.10.1037/0033-295X.111.2.486.

Nentwich, J.C. & Morison, T. (2018). Performing the self: Performativity and discursive psychology. In S.L. Cook, A. Rutheford, C.B. Travis, W.S. Williams, & K.F. Wyche (Eds.), *APA handbook of the psychology of women: History, theory and battlegrounds* (pp. 209–228). Washington, DC: American Psychological Association. https://doi.org/10.1037/0000059-000.

Oyserman, D., Elmore, K., & Smith, G. (2012). Self, self-concept and identity. In M. R. Leary & J.P. Tangney (Eds.), *Handbook of self and identity* (pp. 69–104). New York: The Guildford Press.

Potter, J. & Wetherell, M. (1987). *Discourse and social psychology: Beyond attitudes and behaviour*. London: Sage.

Santamaría, A. & Montoya, E. (2008). La memoria autobiográfica: el encuentro entre la memoria, el yo y el lenguaje. *Estudios de Psicología*, 29(3), 333–350. http://dx.doi.org/10.1174/021093908786145430.

Santamaría, A., Cubero, M., Prados, M., & de la Mata, M.L. (2013). Posiciones y voces ante el cambio coeducativo: la construcción de la identidad del profesorado en la aplicación de planes de igualdad. *Profesorado: Revista de curriculum y formación del profesorado*, 17(1), 28–41.

Shweder, R.A. & Bourne, E.J. (1984). Does the concept of the person vary cross-culturally? In R.A. Shweder & R.A. Levine (Eds.), *Culture theory: Essays on mind, self and emotion* (pp. 158–199). New York: Cambridge University Press.

Swann, W.B. & Bosson, J.K. (2010). Self and identity. In S.T. Fiske, D.T. Gilbert, & G. Lindzey (Eds.), *Handbook of social psychology*, Vol. 1 (5th Edition) (pp. 589–628). Hoboken: Wiley.

Tajfel, H. & Turner, J.C. (1986). The social identity theory of intergroup behaviour. In S. Worchel & W.G. Austin (Eds.), *Psychology of intergroup relations* (pp. 7–24). Chicago: Nelson Hall.

Vignoles, V.T., Schwartz, S.J., & Luyckx, K. (2012). Introduction: Toward an integrative view of identity. In S.J. Schwartz, K. Luyckx, & V.T. Vignoles (Eds.), *Handbook of identity theory and research* (pp. 1–27). New York: Springer-Verlag.

Vygotsky, L.S. (1978). *Mind in society: The development of higher psychological processes*. Cambridge, MA: Harvard University Press.

Wertsch, J.V. (1985). *Vygotsky and the social formation of mind*. Cambridge, MA: Cambridge University Press.

Wertsch, J.V. (1991). *Voices of the mind: A sociocultural approach to mediated action*. Cambridge, MA: Harvard University Press.

Wetherell, M. (2010). The field of identity studies. In M. Wetherell & C.T. Mohanty (Eds.), *The Sage handbook of identities*. Thousand Oaks: SAGE Publications.

Wiggins, S. & Potter, J. (2008). Discursive psychology. In C. Willig & W. Stainton Rogers (Eds.), *The Sage handbook of qualitative research in psychology* (pp. 72–89). London: Sage.

3 Stories of self when living with aphasia in a digitalized society

Helena Taubner, Malin Hallén and Åsa Wengelin

Introduction

The stories we tell about ourselves constitute an interface between us and others. Within this interface, those *stories of self* form our identities as we "keep our narratives going" (Giddens, 1991). This way, identity and language are closely intertwined since we use our linguistic abilities to tell our stories. What happens, then, if a person suddenly loses large parts of his or her language, i.e. acquires *aphasia*, due to a brain injury? Keeping a story of self going requires a certain level of *narrative agency*, i.e. a person's "capacity to make sense of herself as an 'I' over time and in relation to other 'I's" (Lucas, 2017, p. 123). In addition, narrative agency is "the ability and opportunity to author one's own narrative" (Baldwin, 2005, p. 1023), i.e. a combination of the individual linguistic capacities ("ability") and social structures ("opportunity") required to tell stories of self. Without a certain level of narrative agency, our stories of self cannot be told, since it is a "precondition for identity formation" (Lucas, 2017, p. 123). So, when someone acquires aphasia, what becomes of their narrative agency, their stories of self and consequently of themselves? In this chapter, stories of self authored by people (in particular one young woman) with post-stroke aphasia are presented and analysed.

People with aphasia have lost linguistic abilities overnight due to an acquired brain injury (Papathanasiou, Coppens, & Davidson, 2017). Although the variation in severity is large between individuals (Pedersen, Vinter, & Olsen, 2004), they all have the sudden language loss in common. Aphasia may affect talking and listening as well as reading and writing (Johansson-Malmeling, Hartelius, Wengelin, & Henriksson, 2020), but possibly no other aspects of the person's intellect. In this sense, aphasia "masks inherent competence" (Kagan & Simmons-Mackie, 2013) because persons with aphasia may have relatively intact intellectual abilities but the aphasia is "masking" their competence so that they cannot express their thoughts. Since language is central to identity construction, and since narrative agency is essential to author stories of self, acquiring aphasia entails a need of identity re-negotiation (Corsten, Konradi, Schimpf, Hardering, & Keilmann, 2014; Shadden, 2005; Shadden, Hagstrom, & Koski, 2008). People with aphasia have to decide whether to embrace or reject an identity as being disabled (Watson, 2002), i.e. decide whether to include aphasia in their new stories of self or not. To make such a decision, they need to be able to manage certain stigma symbols (Goffman, 1963) such as non-fluent speech or misspellings. Taubner, Hallén, and Wengelin (2017) have shown that people with aphasia in various ways manage such stigma symbols across three dimensions: content, composition and context – or in the words of Kress (2003) "that which is to be communicated" (content), "the modal realisation of the same" (composition), and "the site of appearance" (context).

In addition, someone who experiences a biographical disruption (Bury, 1982) such as acquiring a brain injury may need to navigate certain identity dilemmas; the constancy/change dilemma, the sameness/difference dilemma, and the agency/dependency dilemma (Bamberg, 2011; Glintborg, 2015). Previous research (Taubner, Hallén, & Wengelin, 2020) has shown that people with aphasia do navigate these dilemmas in a constant struggle about what to include in their stories of self. As a result, those stories are filled with contradictions. The studied participants (Taubner et al., 2020) told stories in which they simultaneously were the same as before they acquired aphasia and yet changed (constancy/change), in which they were similar to others (e.g. other stroke survivors or "normal" people) and yet different from them (sameness/difference), and in which they displayed both power and weakness (the agency/dependency dilemma). Additionally, the dilemmas were intertwined, constructing a complex narrative identity.

Not only do people who have acquired aphasia need to author new stories of self in which the aphasia is taken into account – they also have to take on that challenge without their former linguistic capacity. In terms of narrative agency, their ability to author their own narrative is reduced at a time when they would need a high level of narrative agency to process the trauma of having acquired a brain injury. Their key to the identity re-negotiation, i.e. their language, has been reduced when most needed (Shadden et al., 2008). The situation for people with aphasia is, therefore, significantly different from those with disabilities or illnesses that do not include linguistic difficulties (see e.g. Lam & Wodchis, 2010). It is thus of great importance to include issues of language when studying identity and disability. As put by Shadden et al. (2008, p. 14): "we need to understand better the impact of the loss of communication facility at a time when it is most needed to carry on the work of maintaining narrative self".

The language we use to tell our stories of self does not only include spoken words. Not least does it include different forms of writing, an activity which during recent decades has become increasingly digitalized. At the time this chapter is published, almost the entire Swedish population are internet users. For example, 98% have internet access in their homes and 95% own a smartphone (Swedish Internet Foundation, 2019). In such a highly digitalized society, multimodal online literacy practices – i.e. digitalized communication practices based on texts – are central to everyday communication (Barton & Lee, 2013). Texts are no longer merely a set of letters printed on a paper or on a screen. Rather, digital texts include of a large variety of modalities such as links, emoticons, sounds, pictures, videos, or illustrations – i.e. they are based on *multimodality* (Kress, 2010). Navigating this digitalized and multimodal communication landscape has become part of our lifestyles and identities. We have grown accustomed to combining various ways to communicate, including e.g. posting carefully selected pictures on social media (see e.g. Forsman, 2017), sharing links to online newspaper articles, texting messages based on emoticons, and using Google to search for quick answers to almost anything – and people with aphasia are no exception (Taubner, 2019). As a consequence of this digitalization, identity is "always online" (Cover, 2015) and the stories of self told by people living in Sweden – including people with aphasia – will include online aspects.

The aim of this chapter is to analyse stories of self authored by Swedish individuals with post-stroke aphasia, and to discuss the role played by multimodal online literacy practices when telling these stories. The stories of self of one participant in particular (here named Rosa) is used to illustrate the findings.

Method

In order to explore stories of self authored by people with aphasia, nine participants with aphasia were interviewed and observed online (see also Taubner et al., 2017, 2020). All data collection was conducted by the first author. Ethical approval was granted by the Ethical Review Board in Lund, Sweden (ref 2015/109). The nine participants were aged between 24 and 56 when they acquired aphasia, and at the time of their respective interview they were between 29 and 61. Three of them were male and the remaining six were female. When their stories are told below, their names have been replaced with aliases: Rosa, Ellen, Monica, Oskar, Einar, Malin, Frida, Johan and Sofia.

First, so-called Problem-Centred Interviews (Witzel & Reiter, 2012), or PCIs, were conducted face-to-face individually with each participant. This interview method aims at reconstructing knowledge about a relevant topic (a *problem*) and it was chosen because of its focus on the participant's "right to be understood" (Witzel & Reiter, 2012, p. 82). The PCI procedure is based on shifting between questions aimed to generate storytelling and comprehension. Such an approach is suitable when interviewing people with language difficulties, not least for ethical reasons, since it endorses the flexibility needed to meet the communicative needs of the participants. This approach may be seen as a contrast to the frequent exclusion of people with aphasia from research about e.g. strokes or other acquired brain injuries (Townend, Brady, & McLaughlan, 2007). We argue that it is ethically questionable to exclude people with aphasia, and that it is up to us as researchers to adapt our methods in order to include them (Brady, Fredrick, & Williams, 2013; Dalemans, Wade, van den Heuvel, & de Witte, 2009; Pearl & Cruice, 2017). Adaptations are especially important when conducting qualitative research aiming at listening to people's stories – people with aphasia have the right to be listened to despite of their linguistic difficulties. On the other hand, there is a risk of oversimplifying and thus diminishing the person with aphasia. While it is not ethically correct to exclude people with aphasia based on their difficulties, it is also incorrect to, for example, talk exaggeratedly slow (Simmons-Mackie, 2018). In this study, the participants had access to communication aids of their choice. The interviews were conducted at a time and a place suggested by each participant and they lasted between one and three hours. Great effort was made to build trust between the participant and the interviewer (the first author) and to ensure the ease and consent of each participant.

Then, after each interview, observations inspired by "nethnograpy", i.e. ethnographic research based on online fieldwork (Kozinets, 2015), were conducted to collect online data from the participants in social media. Screenshots were captured for online posts made by the participants, mainly on Facebook and Instagram. These nethnographic observations were conducted using a retrospective or archival approach (Kozinets, 2015), which means that the researcher "went back in time" to include data created before and up until the time of the interview. In this way, the collected data has a high level of authenticity since the participants were not influenced by being part of the study when they created the posts. In addition, it was a time-efficient way of collecting data, since data from a large time frame could be collected rapidly. In total, 1,581 screenshots were collected (see also Taubner et al., 2017, 2020). One of the participants, Johan, had no accounts in any observable online network and his online communication activities was limited to professional e-mails. His employer wouldn't permit access to his e-mails, so for ethical reasons no online data was collected. But since his interview provided important information, he is still included in the analysis.

Collecting research data online raises a range of new ethical questions, not least addressed by the Association of Internet Researchers (AoIR) Ethics Working Committee (Markham & Buchanan, 2012). Research ethics as we know it must be revisited to fit online settings. When collecting online data for this study, we have made a number of ethical considerations which deserve some further elaboration. First, there is the question of selecting an online forum to study. Whether or not an online forum is suitable for data collection is a matter of how open the forum is, i.e. whether or not it may be seen as a public space (Sveningsson Elm, 2008). Or in the words of Zimmer (2010, p. 323): "just because personal information is made available in some fashion on a social network, does not mean it is fair game for capture and release to all". The participants were members of a few Facebook groups for stroke survivors or people with aphasia. But, since these groups were deemed semi-closed or in some cases even closed, and since it was not possible to obtain consent from each forum member, these forums were excluded from the data collection. Instead, we only included the participants' posts which were visible as their Facebook "friend" without being part of any Facebook group. When relevant online forums have been selected, consent must be obtained for each specific forum (Baker, 2013), since practices, norm systems, and conventions vary across forums. Agreeing to being observed on Facebook does not necessarily imply agreeing to being observed on a dating site, for instance. For the present study, the participants had the choice to give their consent for each specific forum.

Next, there is the question of anonymity (see e.g. Israel, 2015; Zimmer, 2010). The names and other personal information of the participants were anonymized, and as suggested by Kozinets (2015) this anonymization also included online aliases (e.g. Instagram handles). The question of anonymity is also affected by the privacy settings of the researcher's profile (Baker, 2013). If the relationship between the researcher and the participant is visible to others, the fact that the participant is taking part in the study may be revealed. To avoid these kinds of revealing incidents, the first author created entirely new accounts with maximum security settings to collect the online data. Related to anonymity is the question of protecting third parties, which may seem straightforward but in fact it may not be clear who the third party is. For instance, if a participant is mentioned in someone else's post, and the participant's friends get to see the post because of the "tag", or if a participant shares a post written by someone else – who is the sender of the post and who is the third party? On one hand, every person included in the data collection should have the possibility to give (or decline to give) their consent. On the other hand, it is almost impossible to study communication or interaction without including third-party communicators (Alderson & Morrow, 2011). To sum up this discussion about online research ethics, an awareness that online settings raise new ethical questions is needed from the researcher's part. In this sense, it is beneficial (if not crucial) for the researchers to be familiar with the forums under study, in order to be sensitive to codes, norms, and conventions (Zimmer, 2010). All three authors are active Internet and social media users, which undoubtedly facilitated this study.

The collected material contains a large number of stories of self authored by the nine participants. There is, of course, more to each story than could be fitted into a chapter like this. But we agree with Bamberg and Georgakopoulou (2008) who suggest that even "small stories" may be useful to discuss and analyse narrative identity. Therefore, one participant in particular (here named Rosa), and a set of "small stories" related to her, is used to illustrate the complexity of the ongoing identity re-negotiation when living with aphasia. The other participants' stories are used to mirror – either by confirming or contradicting – Rosa's accounts. Some of the stories have previously been published more extensively. (Taubner et al., 2017, 2020). Each of Rosa's quotes have been translated from Swedish to English, with an intention of imitating her specific linguistic style and ability.

Results

Rosa was 25 years old when she had a stroke, which eventually resulted in aphasia. She could not move nor speak and she knew something was wrong. She was taken to the hospital but it took several days before the medical staff realized that she was in fact having a stroke.

> Rosa: Like, it was bloody awful, you know, I know that something is wrong, but … I couldn't … like, stand up, I couldn't do anything, so I just lay there

> like … And then I woke up … Nobody understood that I was having a stroke, you know (Taubner et al., 2020).

Rosa's physical condition is not very affected by the stroke, but she can feel her face being asymmetric due to right side hemiparesis. Although the hemiparesis is minimal and probably rarely noticeable to others, she is worried that it will show. She doesn't like people staring at her, but when meeting people she often feels that they look at her in a judgemental way. Although she is fully ambulant and her appearance does not imply that she is a stroke survivor, she is afraid that people will judge her based on how she looks. But, simultaneously, she is also aware that she looks "healthy" enough to constantly have to tell people about her difficulties because they are not very visible.

When the stroke occurred, Rosa was a student. Now, because of her fatigue and aphasia, she is not able to neither study nor work, and she has no particular plans for the future. She describes her aphasia in terms of knowing what to say but being unable to say it:

> Rosa: … you KNOW that you can speak, because it's like, kinda, it comes, like and just works kinda. And then when it doesn't WORK … well, it is in here [points to her head]. But not here [points to her mouth] … It is hard to accept, you know.

As a result, Rosa finds it difficult to interact with new people. She says she used to be outspoken and social, but the aphasia has made her feel uncomfortable around new people:

> Rosa: Yeah, well like, you have to like … it makes me really nervous and stuff like, new people, I think, yuk that's hard. New people, ouch!
> Interviewer: Has it always been like that?
> Rosa: No … I love meeting new people, very social, very, like outspoken and like really … so, in that way it is hard. I think it is really hard to meet new people.
> Interviewer: Why has it become like this, you think?
> Rosa: Because I can't speak. Well, I can speak … [sigh].

She concludes that her difficulties meeting new people is caused by her aphasia, saying "I can't speak", but then she also says "Well, I can speak …". She seems to be struggling with how to describe her linguistic abilities and disabilities. On one hand, she cannot speak the way that she used to. On the other hand, she is still able to speak to some extent (not least good enough to be able to participate in the interview). Several of the other participants also express difficulties meeting new people. Sofia, for instance, describes how people sometimes talk to her in a diminishing way. She thus prefers meeting new people online, because it is easier for her to interact there (Taubner et al., 2020).

Another aspect of interacting with other people is that Rosa (as well as the other participants) has to meet their expectations. She says that "everybody" put pressure on her to be strong, but when she is at home alone she sometimes cries and feels weak:

> Rosa: Everybody keeps saying that I am so damn strong and stuff, and then you, then you kinda have to live up to everything they said, and then you get very like … I want to be weak sometimes, too, and such, sometimes it is really hard to be weak and to cry and such, but yeah … when I'm home/when I'm alone, then like …

When Rosa elaborates on her thoughts about her speech being changed, she adds that she feels slower now. She does not understand jokes told by her friends because she is not quick enough, leading to her feeling boring and uncomfortable. She says – and the same thing is expressed by Frida (Taubner et al., 2020) – that she used to be a fun person, but that she cannot be fun any longer:

> Rosa: There was this party, last Saturday … and … then you get so bloody nervous, like even though I know them, it is still hard … Like, I have been a very like fun … a fun person, you know, which I am not today. And that's … this speed, sort of. Because of this, I turn very like, it is really really really hard. It is also a loss, because I don't understand like "yeah but hehe" but I don't get it, but then like [sigh]. And then I'm like "ahaaaa", you know, like that. But I may not even understand, maybe.
> Interviewer: No, I see. It is like you miss out on the jokes?
> Rosa: Yes, sometimes it's like the joke, and then ME, and then … It is hard too. Because I am not very quick any more, today (Taubner et al., 2020).

Feeling slow is an experience that Rosa shares with Johan. He too expresses how his aphasia makes it hard for him to keep up with a conversation, especially if there are many people involved (Taubner et al., 2020).

Aphasia not only entails difficulties speaking (and listening), but possibly also writing (and reading). Even before her stroke, Rosa had difficulties writing, and she says she has "diff- and hm-hm troubles" (referring to reading and writing difficulties). But her former difficulties differ from those related to her aphasia. She says she earlier used to make a few mistakes which are very common to many Swedes, such as confusing the use of the pronouns "de" (they) and "dem" (them) which are both pronounced "dom". But now, she finds it much harder to write, on a more general level. Before her stroke, Rosa used to write poetry, but she cannot do that any longer:

> Rosa: It is called something when you, I used to kinda write really really much, like texts, poty/porety, and such … But yes, well, I used to write REALLY much, so I miss that, writing and such …

Nevertheless, she does communicate a lot in writing. She has accounts on a few different social media forums, of which she mainly uses Facebook. When writing, she prefers to use her smartphone because of the built-in word prediction software. Unfortunately, her smartphone is now broken and to write she must use her computer or her tablet. She finds it more difficult because of the reduced access to supportive tools like the word prediction.

> Rosa: And this [smartphone] is so DAMN good, kinda, when I, so I don't have to kinda think how to, like e … a/c/t [pretends that she is spelling a word], yeah well like that, kinda. Then I just find, kinda, and that amazing … But now [when the smartphone is broken] I really have to, like, SPELL and so on, and shit that's hard. And you just think, no, shit this is hard, but … well it works sort of, but I find it easier to have this [smartphone].

Like Rosa, Malin also relies on technological tools such as word prediction software when writing. But she, in contrast, prefers the one installed on her computer over using her phone. There is a variety among the online writing strategies of the other participants. On one end, there is Oskar who types short and insufficient sentences without any ambition to conceal his aphasia (Taubner et al. 2017). There is also Frida who uses Facebook as a platform for raising awareness about stroke and aphasia (Taubner et al. 2017). On the other end, there is Monica who only posts photos (on Instagram) from a first-person perspective with very short captions. Her posts do not imply that she has aphasia at all (Taubner et al. 2017). Rosa places herself somewhere in between Oskar and Monica when she posts correctly written, although colloquial, texts which occasionally contain content about stroke and aphasia. She does not try to conceal her aphasia, but on the other hand she does not want it to be too visible either.

Rosa's stories of self are complex, not least when it comes to the constancy/change dilemma, i.e. the question of whether she is the same person as she was before her stroke or not. On one hand, she says she is a different and better person now but on the other hand she says that she grieves her old self. During the interview, which takes place one-and-a-half years after her stroke, Rosa says that she is definitely not the same person as before her stroke – that "it's like day and night". Rosa even says she is a better person now (as does Frida), after the stroke, and that her life is better. If she had to choose, she would choose her new life (and self) over the former. She had been using drugs and the stroke gave her an opportunity to become clean, which she now treasures.

> Rosa: Well, it's … I am not the same person, like … it's like day and night.
> Interviewer: In what way?
> Rosa: Well, eh … Yeah, well … I … well, I am a HAPPY person. I have never been grateful and like, I mean for life and such … but I think in a different way today than before. Before the stroke, well … yeah, like … I

> have been an addict and such. No, so I am not, I am not like how it was before or how I was. It seems so damn strange and like … or how to put it.

In fact, Rosa says she is so different now that her former self is dead, and that she – despite being a better person now – grieves her lost self:

> Rosa: Well, it's like this, well, loneliness, like, and sadness. Yes, it is. It is very very much sadness. It's like [Rosa] will never again well, well … well, the old [Rosa], she is dead you know. That's a loss too, you know. And the talking and … So damn much has, has kind of changed and so on, it's like that.

Among the other participants, only Einar and Johan state being the same person as before. They are also the only ones still working in their former professions (Taubner et al., 2020). Both Ellen and Frida also express grief over their lost pre-stroke selves (Taubner et al., 2020).

Rosa's post-stroke self is so different to her pre-stroke self that she is planning on changing her names (both first and surname). But because of her fatigue and aphasia she finds it hard to contact the authorities, and she has not yet gone through the administrative process of changing her names yet. As a consequence, she still, for example, has her old name on her front door. On Facebook, on the other hand, Rosa has created a new profile using her intended new name. The stories presented on her new profile include being a stroke survivor and having aphasia (for example manifested in pictures of her in the hospital bed or of her damaged brain from her medical record), although she mostly posts content about other topics. Her posts often contain a picture or a link and a small caption, mostly written in a relaxed and colloquial way. She uses a lot of emoticons, such as smileys and hearts, to complement her written texts.

Rosa carefully selects which information and pictures of herself to post on Facebook – as does Frida who makes a clear distinction about what to post about her stroke and aphasia on Facebook and on a dating site. On Facebook Frida tells a detailed story about being a stroke survivor, but on the dating site she leaves out all information about her brain injury (Taubner et al. 2017). Rosa posts a lot of selfies on Facebook, in which she wears make up and nice clothes and she looks into the camera which she holds slightly above her face. But she avoids looking cheerful and carefully chooses camera angles, in order to conceal her (minimal) hemiparesis. This strategy is shared with Ellen, who also avoids smiling in her Facebook pictures in order to conceal her slightly lopsided face. In photos where others are seen with a big smile, Ellen's smile is much more modest. Ellen says she chooses photos in which she looks good, excluding photos in which she is smiling because her asymmetric smile would reveal her hemiparesis and make her feel ugly. Her friends sometimes remark on her never smiling in her selfies, implying that they think she looks boring. Thus, both Ellen and Rosa seem to prefer to be perceived as boring or unhappy (i.e. not smiling) over ugly (i.e. with a lopsided face), and hence they conceal their smiles when posting selfies. Additionally, Rosa makes a clear distinction between her stroke and a heart condition of hers. Because of this heart condition, she has a post-surgery scar along her sternum, which she (in contrast to her asymmetrical smile) occasionally proudly displays in her selfies. Thus, she seems to wear her heart surgery scar with pride, but feels ashamed of her stroke:

> Rosa: I … like, I am not ashamed over things like this [points at the scar from her heart surgery]. No but you think it is like it has to look good, like, obviously … when I smile and such like, you have to kinda … So, so if you look, like you really can see it [that the face is lopsided] if you really look at me like. Of course, I want to look good, you know.

Posting photos on a Facebook wall is an asynchronous activity, but Facebook also provides a possibility of interacting synchronously by using Messenger for chatting. Rosa says she and her friends do chat on Messenger, but that she gets tired when the conversations get too long. She tried to tell her friends, but it seems to her like they do not understand and instead she makes up white lies to end the conversation:

> Interviewer: Do you and your friends use Messenger to chat?
> Rosa: Eh, yes, we do. Yes, we do. But mostly kinda … well yeah, but like, I, well, I kinda choose. If I don't want to, I can, you see, when it gets long and like … Sometimes I feel like they never will understand. That's what's hard. So you try to make a like, a white lie, instead of telling them the truth.

In a similar way, Einar avoids using synchronous tools such as Messenger because he finds it hard to write at an anticipated speed and pace (Taubner et al. 2017). He also avoids writing by instead using the "like-button" on Facebook, which gives him an opportunity to engage in communication with his friends and show them his presence, without having to actually write (Taubner et al. 2017).

To conclude, Rosa's stories of self are complex and contradicting and they vary across all three dimensions of composition ("the modal realisation"), content ("that which is to be communicated") and context ("the site of appearance"). They, for instance, depend on who she is interacting with, what tools she has access to and whether she is communicating online or offline. Online she uses a large variety of tools and modalities (photos, emoticons, links, etc.) which are not available to her when interacting offline. This range of modalities gives her an opportunity to choose how to compose her stories of self (e.g. how to arrange her selfies or which emoticons to include in a caption) in different contexts, and this in turn makes it possible for her to choose the content of her stories (i.e. whether or not to include being a stroke survivor with aphasia). In fact, the online settings even provide her with an opportunity to start a completely new story of self under a new name.

Discussion

The stories of self authored by Rosa (and the other participants) show that her (as well as the others') ongoing identity re-negotiation is complex. Her stories include various contradictions, which shows that she does recurrently negotiate what to include in her stories of self (see also Taubner et al., 2017) and that she constantly navigates identity dilemmas (see also Taubner et al., 2020). She tells stories of self in which she makes a clear distinction between her pre- and post-stroke self. She says that she used to be an outspoken and social person who loved to meet new people. She was a fun person who was quick enough to make and understand jokes. She was a person who wrote poetry. Neither of these aspects are included in her stories about her present post-stroke self. Now she is instead shy and reserved when meeting new people, and she misses out on people's jokes, resulting in stories of self which are about being asocial and boring. And although she had writing difficulties before her stroke, she says she is now completely unable to write poetry. In fact, she makes such a clear distinction between who she was before and who she is now that she talks about her pre-stroke self as being dead and that she is planning to change her names. But she has not gone through that process yet, meaning that she is still officially identified by her old name. On the other hand, she has created a new Facebook profile in which she uses her new intended name. Thus, offline she is in some ways still perceived as the same person as before the stroke, but online she tells a completely new story. Similarly, the other participants also author stories of self about both being the same as they were pre-stroke and changed; they are both the same and different in relation to others, i.e. both "disabled" and "normal"; they display both dependency and agency (see also Taubner et al., 2020).

Rosa describes her new self as happier and more grateful than she was before (but on the other hand she also says that she grieves her pre-stroke self). The main reason for this big change is that the stroke gave Rosa an opportunity to leave her drug addiction behind and become clean. She thus prefers her new self even with the aphasia and other consequences of the stroke. When communicating online (mainly on Facebook using her new profile) that is the story she tells, i.e. about being sober but also being a stroke survivor with aphasia. She uses technological tools to compensate for her writing difficulties (as a way to manage stigma symbols) and she writes in a colloquial way which is socially anticipated way when writing on Facebook. She chooses very carefully how to present herself in her selfies – stating that she wants to look good – making a difference between her post-surgery scar (which she proudly displays) and her slightly lopsided face (which she conceals by not smiling). Thus, although she is grateful for her post-stroke self, she is also ashamed over how the stroke has changed her appearance and she chooses to conceal the stigma symbols which could reveal her aphasia and hemiparesis. She thus conceals her disabilities in the composition dimensions but reveals it regarding content. She may therefore be perceived both as a person *with* and *without* aphasia and other consequences of her stroke, which is an example of how she navigates the sameness/difference dilemma (Bamberg, 2011) – and it becomes clear that navigation of the dilemmas and stigma management are closely related.

The short comparisons to the other participants show that there is a variety of strategies, even in such a small sample as this. As a way to navigate the constancy/change dilemma (Bamberg, 2011), some of the participants (including Rosa) mainly focus on being changed, while others tells stories about being the same (mainly Einar and Johan, who also are the only ones who work in their pre-stroke professions), and in addition each story contains contradictions. The participants tell stories in which they are both the same and different in relation to others (Bamberg, 2011), i.e. both "disabled" and "normal". They simultaneously embrace and reject a disability identity (Watson, 2002). In Rosa's story, this sameness/difference dilemma is manifested in her constant concerns about other people's perceptions of her. She is worried that they will judge her based on her looks – even though the physical consequences of her stroke are barely visible. She is grateful and proud of being a stroke survivor with aphasia, but at the same time she does not want people to judge her based on her disabilities. This concern leads her to arrange her Facebook selfies in a way that her hemiparesis is less visible. She thus tells a story in which she presents herself as both "disabled" (mainly in the content of her communication) and "normal" (mainly in the composition of her communication). She does not want others to draw any conclusions about her (dis)abilities based on what they see, but she wants to tell them when and how she chooses to herself. Rosa is not unique when it comes to selecting very carefully how to be portrayed in online photos. As mentioned, Ellen shares her experiences and strategies, but they are also both part of a society in which young women are expected to look and behave in certain ways online (Forsman, 2017). A third dilemma is that the stories contained both dependency and agency (Bamberg, 2011). For instance, Rosa expresses an expectation from others that she should be strong, but that she also wants to be allowed to feel weak. This may be one reason that she sometimes makes up white lies to end (chat) conversations with her friends. They expect her to be strong, so she prefers telling them that she has to go over telling them that she feels weak.

The "small stories" (Bamberg & Georgakopoulou, 2008) presented in this chapter highlight that linguistic aspects have to be taken into account when studying identity and disability. The complexity of Rosa's (and the others participants') stories of self are highly influenced by the aphasia. For example, she finds it hard to interact with new people because of her difficulties speaking. She feels slow and boring when she cannot keep up with their jokes. Consequently, she cannot present herself as the person she wants to (and used to) be. She says she used to be "a fun person, you know, which I am not today", meaning that others get a picture of her that differs from her own idea of who she wants to be. The experience of being slow and thus being perceived as boring or distant is shared with Frida, Johan, and Ellen. Not only do they have to tell new stories of self in which they navigate being stroke survivors with aphasia, they also have to author these new stories while feeling unable to communicate in an anticipated way. Their language is lost "when most needed" (Shadden et al., 2008). Another example is that Rosa also describes herself as a person who used to write very much, including poetry, but who is now unable to write (although she actually writes a lot on Facebook, for example). This is clearly a linguistic aspect of her stories of self, since literacy practices are an important part of telling these stories. She struggles with the anticipated speed and pace when writing synchronously (i.e. chatting) with her friends, and instead of telling them about her difficulties she makes up white lies to end the conversation. Thus, she prefers to be not completely honest with her friends over revealing her disabilities. In these situations, she tells stories of self that does not include aphasia because she does not believe her friends would understand.

The chapter aims not only to analyse stories of self, but also to discuss the role played by multimodal online literacy practices when telling these stories. Throughout Rosa's stories, it becomes clear that those practices are important to her ongoing identity re-negotiation. She is part of a highly digitalized society in which multimodal literacy practices are central (Barton & Lee, 2013) and in which identity is always online (Cover, 2015). Through their large variety of modalities, these online literacy practices provide opportunities for her to author her own narratives despite her difficulties – i.e. they increase her narrative agency (Baldwin, 2005; Lucas, 2017). Overall, the findings show that because of the multimodality, the online literacy practices provide an opportunity for the participants to express their stories of self in a more elaborate way than in offline settings (Taubner et al., 2017, 2020). When communicating through for instance Facebook, Instagram, or e-mail, the wide range of modalities (such as the possibility to post photos, videos, illustrations or emoticons, or to press a like-button) provides an opportunity to choose tools that compensate some of the difficulties of each individual. They may to a higher extent choose to communicate in ways that conceal or reveal their difficulties, depending on their abilities, intentions, and ambitions. Whether a person with aphasia wants to tell a story of self which include the linguistic difficulties or not, they may find ways to do so when being involved in multimodal online literacy practices.

Narrative agency requires both abilities (on an individual level) and opportunities (on a social level) to author one's own narrative (Baldwin, 2005; Lucas, 2017) and aphasia entails reduced linguistic abilities. But multimodal online literacy practices, found for instance on Facebook or Instagram, increase the opportunities for people with aphasia to author their own narrative, more than offline and less multimodal practices do. When the opportunities increase, in ways that may compensate for the person's impaired abilities, so does the narrative agency and hence also the possibility to author stories of self. In other words, the large variety of modalities provided by online platforms such as Facebook or Instagram gives people with aphasia an opportunity to tell their stories of self despite their individual difficulties. They can choose how to navigate identity dilemmas, how to manage stigma symbols and whether to embrace or reject an identity as "being disabled". Without the multimodality, their stories would not be as rich or complex because they would not have these options. The point is not that the participants choose to tell stories which displays their aphasia (and other aspects of being a stroke survivor) or not, but that they – when being engaged in multimodal online literacy practices – get to make that choice. The online multimodality provides an opportunity to show just how complex the stories of self are when living with aphasia.

References

Alderson, P. & Morrow, V. (2011). *The ethics of research with children and young people: A practical handbook*, Vol. 2. Los Angeles: SAGE.

Baker, S. (2013). Conceptualising the use of Facebook in ethnographic research: As tool, as data and as context. *Ethnography and Education*, 8(2), 131–145. doi:10.1080/17457823.2013.792504.

Baldwin, C. (2005). Narrative, ethics and people with severe mental illness. *Australian and New Zealand Journal of Psychiatry*, 39(11–12), 1022–1029. doi:10.1080/j.1440-1614.2005.01721.x.

Bamberg, M. (2011). Who am I? Narration and its contribution to self and identity. *Theory & Psychology*, 21(1), 3–24. doi:10.1177/0959354309355852.

Bamberg, M. & Georgakopoulou, A. (2008). Small stories as a new perspective in narrative and identity analysis. *Text & Talk*, 28(3), 377–396.

Barton, D. & Lee, C. (2013). *Language online: Investigating digital texts and practices.* Oxford: Routledge.

Brady, M.C., Fredrick, A., & Williams, B. (2013). People with aphasia: Capacity to consent, research participation and intervention inequalities. *International Journal of Stroke*, 8(3), 193–196. doi:10.1111/j.1747-4949.2012.00900.x.

Bury, M. (1982). Chronic illness as biographical disruption. *Sociology of Health and Illness*, 4(2), 167–182.

Corsten, S., Konradi, J., Schimpf, E.J., Hardering, F., & Keilmann, A. (2014). Improving quality of life in aphasia: Evidence for the effectiveness of the biographic-narrative approach. *Aphasiology*, 28(4), 440–452. doi:10.1080/02687038.2013.843154.

Cover, R. (2015). *Digital identities: Creating and communicating the online self.* London: Academic Press.

Dalemans, R., Wade, D., van den Heuvel, W., & de Witte, L. (2009). Facilitating the participation of people with aphasia in research: A description of strategies. *Clinical Rehabilitation*, 23(10), 948–959. doi:10.1177/0269215509337197.

Forsman, M. (2017). Duckface/stoneface: Selfie stereotypes and selfie literacy in gendered media practices in Sweden. In L. Dafna & G. Maya (Eds.), *Beyond stereotypes? Images of boys and girls, and their consequences* (pp. 193–202). Gothenburg: Nordicom.

Giddens, A. (1991). *Modernity and self-identity: Self and society in the late modern age.* Cambridge: Polity Press.

Glintborg, C. (2015). Disabled and not normal: Identity construction after an acquired brain injury. *Narrative Inquiry*, 25(1), 1–21. doi:10.1075/ni.25.1.01gli.

Goffman, E. (1963). *Stigma: Notes on the management of spoiled identity.* London: Penguin.

Israel, M. (2015). *Research ethics and integrity for social scientists* (2nd Edition). Thousand Oaks: SAGE.

Johansson-Malmeling, C., Hartelius, L., Wengelin, Å., & Henriksson, I. (2020). Written text production and its relationship to writing processes and spelling ability in persons with post-stroke aphasia. *Aphasiology*, 1–18. doi:10.1080/02687038.2020.1712585.

Kagan, A. & Simmons-Mackie, N. (2013). From my perspective: Changing the aphasia narrative. *The ASHA Leader*, 18(11), 6–8. doi:10.1044/leader.FMP.18112013.6.

Kozinets, R.V. (2015). *Netnography: Redefined* (2nd Edition). London: SAGE.

Kress, G. (2003). *Literacy in the new media age*. London: Routledge.

Kress, G. (2010). *Multimodality, a social semiotic approach to contemporary communication*. Oxford: Routledge.

Lam, J.M.C. & Wodchis, W.P. (2010). The relationship of 60 disease diagnoses and 15 conditions to preference-based health-related quality of life in Ontario hospital-based long-term care residents. *Medical Care*, 48(4), 380–387. doi:10.1097/MLR.0b013e3181ca2647.

Lucas, S.D. (2017). The primacy of narrative agency: Re-reading Seyla Benhabib on narrativity. *Feminist Theory*, 19(2), 123–143. doi:10.1177/1464700117723591.

Markham, A.N. & Buchanan, E. (2012). *Ethical decision-making and internet research: Recommendations from the AoIR ethics working committee (version 2.0)*. Chicago: Association of Internet Researchers. Retrieved from: aoir.org/reports/ethics2.pdf.

Papathanasiou, I., Coppens, P., & Davidson, B. (2017). Aphasia and related neurogenic communication disorders: Basic concepts, management, and efficacy. In I. Papathanasiou & P. Coppens (Eds.), *Aphasia and related neurogenic communication disorders* (2nd Edition) (pp. 3–14). Burlington: Jones & Bartlett Learning.

Pearl, G. & Cruice, M. (2017). Facilitating the involvement of people with aphasia in stroke research by developing communicatively accessible research resources. *Topics in Language Disorders*, 37(1), 67–84. doi:10.1097/TLD.0000000000000112.

Pedersen, P.M., Vinter, K., & Olsen, T.S. (2004). Aphasia after stroke: Type, severity and prognosis – the Copenhagen aphasia study. *Cerebrovascular Diseases*, 17(1), 35–43. doi:10.1159/000073896.

Shadden, B. (2005). Aphasia as identity theft: Theory and practice. *Aphasiology*, 19(3–5), 211–223. doi:10.1080/02687930444000697.

Shadden, B., Hagstrom, F. & Koski, P.R. (2008). *Neurogenic communication disorders: Life stories and the narrative self.* San Diego: Plural Publishing.

Simmons-Mackie, N. (2018). Communication partner training in aphasia: Reflections on communication accommodation theory. *Aphasiology*, 32(10), 1215–1224. doi:10.1080/02687038.2018.1428282.

Sveningsson Elm, M. (2008). How do various notions of privacy influence decisions in qualitative internet research? In A.N. Markham & N.K. Baym (Eds.), *Internet inquiry: Conversations about method* (pp. 69–93). Thousand Oaks: SAGE.

Swedish Internet Foundation. (2019). *The Swedes and the internet 2019*. Retrieved from: svenskarnaochinternet.se/English.

Taubner, H. (2019). Increased agency through screens and co-creation: Literacy practices within a group of people with aphasia at a Swedish folk high school. *Scandinavian Journal of Disability Research*, 21(1), 197–206. doi:10.16993/sjdr.635.

Taubner, H., Hallén, M., & Wengelin, Å. (2017). Signs of aphasia: Online identity and stigma management in post-stroke aphasia. *Cyberpsychology: Journal of Psychosocial Research on Cyberspace*, 11(1), article 10. doi:10.5817/CP2017-1-10.

Taubner, H., Hallén, M., & Wengelin, Å. (2020). Still the same? Self-identity dilemmas when living with post-stroke aphasia in a digitalised society. *Aphasiology*, 34(3), 300–318. doi:10.1080/02687038.2019.1594151.

Townend, E., Brady, M., & McLaughlan, K. (2007). Exclusion and inclusion criteria for people with aphasia in studies of depression after stroke: A systematic review and future recommendations. *Neuroepidemiology*, 29(1–2), 1–17. doi:10.1159/000108913.

Watson, N. (2002). Well, I know this is going to sound very strange to you, but I don't see myself as a disabled person: Identity and disability. *Disability & Society*, 17(5), 509–527. doi:10.1080/09687590220148496.

Witzel, A. & Reiter, H. (2012). *The problem-centred interview*. London: SAGE.

Zimmer, M. (2010). "But the data is already public": On the ethics of research in Facebook. *Ethics and Information Technology*, 12(4), 313–325. doi:10.1007/s10676-010-9227-5.

4 "We got a second chance"

Couple narratives after being affected by an acquired brain injury

Chalotte Glintborg and Cecilie M.S. Thøgersen

Worldwide, estimates are that 1 in 50 people will acquire a brain injury in their lifetime (Brain Injury Association of Queensland, 2010). Acquired brain injuries (ABI) are associated with long-term, frequently debilitating symptoms that extend well beyond common physical complications. In fact, symptoms in emotional and social domains are often cited as the ABI complications that create the greatest long-term struggle to successful survivorship (Zasler et al., 2012; Glintborg & Hansen, in press). Thus, worldwide adults with ABI are profoundly impacted by these injuries.

In addition to the chronic, whole-life implications for many individuals currently diagnosed with ABI, clinicians in the field of rehabilitation have long identified ABI as a "family injury" (Lezak, 1988). As such, the emotional and psychological toll of injury on an ABI survivor can be secondary in impact to the deleterious effects on family members and family relationships (Lezak, 1986). Spouses in particular are often negatively impacted. Spousal rates of depression in the years following ABI diagnosis have long been shown to outpace rates of ABI survivor depression (Mauss-Clum & Ryan, 1981). ABI survivors in a committed relationship will rely on their partner to be their caregiver (Brooks, 1991), resulting in substantial caregiver burden, relationship role confusion (Anderson, Parmenter, & Mok, 2002), an unbalancing of responsibilities (Gill, Sander, Robins, Mazzei, & Struchen, 2011), and isolation from sources of social support (Nabors, Seacat, & Rosenthal, 2002).

Long-term outcomes are heavily tied to family well-being after ABI. For example, family functioning is less associated with the degree of injury severity than with the whole-family psychological factors associated with ABI, such as burden, stress, and neurobehavioural functioning (Kreutzer, Gervasio, & Camplair, 1994). In addition, family member functioning is positively correlated with long-term survivor outcomes. Yet neither families nor spouses routinely receive services during acute rehabilitation or as part of long-term postacute rehabilitation. Spouses and family members, who become acculturated into the individually focused medical paradigm, learn to focus all their attention and energy on the medical, physical, emotional, and social care of the ABI survivor. As a result, spouses often struggle to prioritize self-care as well as the care of noninjured family members. Without intervention, the family's pull towards maintaining stability can result in these intensely unbalanced relationships persisting indefinitely.

ABI is classified as a chronic condition (Masel & DeWitt, 2010), rather than an acute injury, because of the enduring nature of physical, emotional, behavioural, and social survivor symptoms and the long-term exacerbated stress levels, social isolation, and sustained emotionality often experienced by the whole family. A decade after injury, family members and survivors continue to report difficulty with emotional and psychological functioning (Seel, Macciocchi, & Kreutzer, 2010), family and marital stability (Kreutzer, Marwitz, Hsu, Williams, & Riddick, 2007), financial security (Carnes & Quinn, 2005), and life satisfaction (Kolakowsky-Hayner, Miner, & Kreutzer, 2001).

Traditionally, research has focused on the negative consequences of ABI. Whilst this is understandable given that six months post-ABI approximately one-third of survivors develop clinically relevant psychological distress (Hackett & Anderson, 2005; Bombardier et al., 2010), the fact that a substantial proportion of people with ABI do not develop psychological distress means that positive and protective mechanisms are also worthy of consideration.

Applying positive psychological principles to ABI rehabilitation is growing, captured in a movement that emphasizes "building what's strong" rather than "fixing what's wrong" (Evans, 2011). Over the past 13 years more people are subscribing to the idea that positive growth may be possible after ABI, particularly when changes occur in relation to a person's sense of meaning, purpose, heightened spirituality, and enhanced relationships after brain injury (Tedeschi & Calhoun, 2004).

Benefit finding, post-traumatic growth, and narratives

Around the turn of the century a paradigm shift occurred in the stress and coping literature with the evolution of a positive psychology approach based on constructs such as adversarial growth and benefit finding (Tennen & Affleck, 2002). This shift had been building for more than 20 years, largely from the work on post-traumatic growth (Linley & Joseph, 2004). There followed a growth in the research literature on benefit finding in chronic illness and disability (Helgeson, Reynolds, & Tomich, 2006), and also among family caregivers (Cassidy, 2012; Cassidy, Giles, & McLaughlin, 2013). Helgeson et al. (2006) identified 235 studies, over half of which had been carried out between 2001 and 2006, and covered a range of chronic illnesses, war, sexual assault, disasters, and having a chronically ill child. Their meta-analysis concluded that benefit finding was related to lower levels of depression and more positive well-being, but was also correlated with more intrusive thoughts and was not correlated with self-rated physical health (Helgeson et al., 2006, p. 810). Individual studies, however, have shown clear links between benefit finding and health. One of the first in the area was conducted by Affleck, Tennen, Croog, and Levine (1987), with 287 men who had recently experienced their first heart attack. Over 50% of men reported benefits and those who did were significantly less likely to have a subsequent heart attack and exhibited lower morbidity rates eight years later, controlling for age, socio-economic status, and disease severity. Bower, Kemeny, Taylor, and Fahey (1998) showed benefit finding to be linked to less rapid decline in health and even reduced mortality in a sample of AIDS sufferers. Similar physiological benefits were shown in cancer patients (McGregor & Antoni, 2009). However, the mechanisms linking benefit finding and health are still unclear (Bower, Moskowitz, & Epel, 2009). Bower et al. (2009) propose what could be described as a resource model of stress to explain the pathways from benefit finding to health, turning the traditional deficit model of stress (Lazarus & Folkman, 1984) on its head. They proposed that benefit finding leads to increased psychological and social resources, through improving coping strategies, thereby making the individual more resilient and less responsive to stressful demands.

The literature has grown and measures have been developed and it appears that most researchers view benefit finding as a multidimensional construct which describes the processes involved in growth or benefit finding rather than just its existence (Tomich & Helgeson, 2004). These authors identified six factors: acceptance, empathy, appreciation, family domain, positive self-view, and reprioritization. It seems more appropriate then to define benefit finding as "the process of growth", and to allow the possibility that it may occur in more everyday settings as well as in response to trauma.

In addition, past research has largely focused on demonstrating the existence of benefit finding following trauma and its relationship with health outcomes, with little or no research on factors that might contribute to or mediate benefit finding (Bower et al., 2009). Only one multidimensional measure is to be found in the literature, the Perceived Benefit Scale (McMillen & Fisher, 1998), which is a 27-item scale measuring eight factors: lifestyle changes, material gain, increases in self-efficacy, family closeness, community closeness, faith in people, compassion, and spirituality.

There is a large and increasing literature on the emotional impact of ABI. This includes systematic accounts of the natural process(es) of psychological adjustment undergone by the survivor, friends, and family; and also, the development of therapeutic approaches to optimize adjustment (see, for instance, Bowen, Yeates, & Palmer, 2010; McGrath & King, 2004; Glintborg, 2015; Glintborg & Hansen, 2016; Glintborg, 2019). The present chapter suggests that the area would be enhanced by the incorporation of the relatively new concept of "post-traumatic growth" (PTG), not least because it offers a psychologically grounded entrée into the area of spirituality in ABI survivors and partners.

Richard Tedeschi and Lawrence Calhoun wrote the book *Trauma and Transformation* in 1995. Tedeschi and Calhoun described the most common benefits reported in the aftermath of trauma as a greater appreciation of life; improved quality of relationships with those going through the same thing, or who have been there to help; a discovery of unexpected personal strengths; the opening up of unforeseen life options; and a deepened "spirituality" (Tedeschi & Calhoun, 1995).

If spirituality is understood as goal-directed transcendence, it can be seen that there is considerable overlap with the concept of PTG. Tedeschi and Calhoun conceive of spirituality as one of the areas in which PTG can occur. PTG involves transcendence of (not the same as dissociation from) a terrible situation, expressed in rearranged priorities and goals, corresponding to "vertical spirituality"; a discovery of previously hidden inner psychological strengths in the context of apparent weakness, corresponding to "interior spirituality"; and an increased sense of connection with other people, corresponding to "horizontal spirituality". The reorientation entailed in establishing a new life path can occasionally occur quite suddenly and dramatically in the aftermath of trauma (Miller & C'de Baca, 2001), and this has been linked with the phenomenon of religious conversion (McIntosh, 1995; Ullman, 1982).

As writers such as Viktor Frankl (1963) and Ronnie Janoff-Bulman (1992) have pointed out, there is an existential heart to trauma. Trauma shatters our core assumptions about the world and ourselves: it assaults us by forcing us to consider the possibility that the world is meaningless, that it is beyond our control, that we are insignificant or even worthless and that our rules for living do not work. "Genuine" PTG is said to occur when these core assumptions have been reinstated in a more sophisticated form, taking the traumatic event into account, so that it comes to occupy a central place in a reconstituted life narrative (Tedeschi & Calhoun, 1995; see also Nochi (2000) for a detailed account of this process in traumatic brain injury (TBI) survivors). So, the cognitive processes that are at work in PTG are focused on the big questions of existential significance that are also the focus of spirituality.

Narratives

McAdams (1993) has conjectured that trauma or crisis provides an opportunity for people to re-create their life narratives and to structure a life story with coherence and meaning. From this perspective, there are individuals who characteristically provide narratives in which misfortune or life tragedy contains a positive aspect or leads to a positive outcome.

In a similar vein *sense-making* denotes the comprehensibility of the loss or the survivor's or partner's capacity to find some sort of benign explanation for the seemingly inexplicable experience, often framed in philosophical or spiritual terms. Conversely, benefit-finding refers to the significance of the loss and entails the survivor's or partner's paradoxical ability to uncover a "silver lining" in the personal or social consequences of the loss, such as enhanced empathy, reordered life priorities, or a closer connection to other people within or beyond the family. Post-traumatic growth involves sense-making. First, the fact that the event happened at all has to be worked through in relation to pre-existing beliefs about justice and order in the world – the "What have I done to deserve this?" question. In his writings on religion as coping, Pargament draws a distinction between two types of religious–spiritual coping: coping that conserves significance and coping that transforms significance (Pargament, 1997).

Methods

In this study, we see couples' narrative identity as being performed in not only a given context, but also within a certain research setting. The story told in a specific research situation cannot be seen as a self-contained product that mirrors a private psychological reality, because it cannot be divorced from the social context from which it originated: the interview situation. The transcribed interview is not seen as strictly monological text, but analysed with reference to the communicative situation of the research interview.

As an approach to narrative identity, this study draws on discursive psychology (Davies & Harré, 1990; Potter & Wetherell, 1987). This means that identity is understood as constructed in discourse, as negotiated among speaking subjects in social contexts, and as emergent. This contrasts with a more traditional view of identity as self-contained (*having* identity) with the consequence that the means by which an individual generates his/her own individuality and character is seen as a personal identity project; here the focus is on the process (De Fina, Schiffrin, & Bamberg, 2006; Bamberg, De Fina, & Schiffrin, 2011). According to Bamberg (2011), any claim of identity will face three dilemmas: (1) successful diachronic navigation between constancy and change; (2) the establishment of a synchronic connection between sameness and difference (between self and other); and (3) the management of agency between the double arrow of a person-to-world versus world-to-person direction fit (Bamberg, 2011, p. 6).

"Dominant discourses" or "master narratives" are taken up in a type of discourse analysis called "positioning theory" (Bamberg, 2003; Bamberg & Georgakopoulou, 2008; Davies & Harré, 1990). Positioning theory refers broadly to the close inspection of how speakers describe people and their actions in one way rather than another and, by doing so, perform discursive actions that result in acts of identity (Davies & Harré, 1990, p. 46).

The data considered in this chapter form part of a larger mixed-method longitudinal five-year follow-up study. Part of this research project consists of semi-structured interviews with adults with ABI. Interviews were chosen as a fruitful method to capture narrations.

A five-year follow-up study was conducted on a cohort of adults with a moderate or severe ABI and their close relatives admitted to the neurorehabilitation centre in the Northern Region of Denmark. The inclusion criteria were: (1) age 18–66 years; (2) residence in Aalborg, Jammerbugt, Vest Himmerland, or Bronderslev municipality; and (3) admission to Bronderslev Neurorehabilitation Center (BNC) in 2013/2014. Forty-five adults met the inclusion criteria. All participants were interviewed three times, after providing informed consent. The first author conducted the three follow-up interviews and a supplementary interview was done by the second author. The first interview took place in the acute phase during hospitalization (year 2013/2014), and the second interview took place one year post-injury (year 2014/2015) and the third interview took place five years post-injury (year 2018/2019). The second and third interviews took place in the informants' own homes. Interviews were recorded and later transcribed.

A thematic content analysis (Braun & Clarke, 2006) on all interviews revealed predominant patterns, reported by almost all of the participants. One of these patterns was post-traumatic growth/resilience and will be explored in depth in this chapter with reference to a single case study. The couple in this single case study are named Lillian and Kenny. To protect participants' anonymity and confidentiality, all identifying details and specifics of the interviews have been altered. Furthermore, the research project has been granted permission by the Danish Data Protection Agency.

The following transcription notation is used:

Bold: informant stresses a word
(.): Short pause
(…): Longer pause
…: a new sentence replaces another (example: It's like when…I mean).

Analysis

Lillian is 63 years old and her husband Kenny is 68 years old when Lillian suffers from three haemorrhage bleedings. Shortly before Lillian's ABI, Kenny was diagnosed with prostate cancer. They have been in a relationship since college and have two adult sons. Both Kenny and Lillian were working at the time they both became ill. Kenny as an accountant and Lillian as a nurse. Lillian did not return to work after her ABI, but Kenny continued to work. They live in a house in a small suburb of a larger Danish city.

Across all four interviews with Kenny and Lillian, spirituality plays an important role in this their narratives. When initially asked about acquiring the brain injury and what happened, spirituality comes up.

A reminder

> K: We did not take it that seriously, because it was shortly after my own diagnosis with prostate cancer (…) We are a bit spiritual both of us, so we took it (…) my wife took it as a reminder. She felt it as a slap in her neck.

A slap in the neck can be an early warning sign of a haemorrhage bleeding. Yet, Lillian connects this "slap" with their current situation and constructs it as a spiritual *reminder* of this. However, one week later, Lillian went to the hospital because she felt sick. She felt nauseous and had a headache. While she was at the hospital, she had another bleeding and went directly into a coma for four months. Luckily, she was at the hospital at the time. The next four months, Lillian is hospitalized and in a coma. Kenny drives two hours every single day to visit Lillian at the hospital. He describes this period of time as extremely hard – even for a former elite soldier:

> K: It was rough. I have never experienced anything this tough. I have been an elite soldier, but this (…) This was worse than I could ever imagine. It was the worst four months. I went to the hospital every single day to see her.

Kenny compares the four months with being a former elite soldier, but the four months were harder. The position of an elite soldier draws on a military discourse of being strong, independent and not sensitive or weak. The elite soldier is capable of going to war to fight or kill and to risk his or her own life.

During these daily visits, Kenny felt a connection with Lillian even though she was in a coma:

> K: I got a feeling that she was not gone. When I entered the hospital room she registered me and she could communicate. I had the feeling that she was inside there underneath the shell (.) but I could not convince the doctors that there was something wrong. They had found a fluid accumulation in the brain – not that big and they observed it so it did not get any bigger. I insisted on a pressure measurement, but they were reluctant to do that (…) Finally, she got it and the day after … no I think it was the same day, they put a valve in her and the day after she opened her eyes and we could talk together. It went so fast.

In this account, we see a conflict between what Kenny senses and what the doctors observe. In other words, there is a conflict between a medical and a spiritual discourse. Kenny felt that there was something wrong, but it was only a sense. He was hopeful and optimistic. This optimism stands in contrast with what the doctors predicted and had Lillian listed up for:

> K: (…) They had recommended a nursing home. She did not respond to their training. I did not feel that she was so ill (…) They did not want to hear that I had contact with her…that was weird. They apparently did not, but I think it was the voice (Kenny's voice).

On top of the fact that Kenny had a wife in coma, he had to struggle to convince the doctors that what he was sensing was true. He was right. However, he is wondering whether her ABI consequences could have been minor if she has gotten the valve sooner.

The medical discourse is also present when Lillian wakes up after four weeks in a coma. She describes herself as being super happy to be alive and she is happy to see Kenny again. "It is like we are falling in love all over again", she says. However, Lillian is told by a neuropsychologist that she seems almost artificially happy, and it is noted in her journal that they (the professionals) must be aware of behavioural changes. Lillian is amazed by this description in the journal, since she really felt happy to be alive at this point.

Because of the enormous power in professional–survivor relations, there is a risk that the professional's interpretations and narratives about a person with ABI can become the truth and the narratives of persons with ABI can be silenced. Silencing people with disabilities through the assertion of the expert's professional opinion occurs routinely, especially in cases of neurological or psychiatric disabilities where insight issues appear and the survivor's personal judgment is considered to be out of play. However, both Kenny and Lillian stood strong in their own beliefs and mindset and challenge the offered positions from professionals.

Daily emails

When Kenny is asked what kept him going in this double struggle, he answers:

> K: The think that kept me going was (…) every day when I got home, I sat down at the computer and sent an email out to family and friends and wrote how the situation was as seen from my perspective.

Kenny is coping with the situation by writing daily emails. Kenny describes that these emails were always written in a very positive and optimistic tone. He got a lot of different feedback on these emails. In this way, he could share the situation with family and friends. However, some thought that he was too optimistic in these emails. For instance, some of Lillian's colleagues thought that these emails were seen from a too optimistic or unrealistic perspective, but as Kenny puts it, "It wasn't".

> L: They [Lillian's colleagues] were so afraid that he was too unrealistic and was in denial and stuff like that because they (…) but it got me through this, honey.
> K: (…) I got air that way (…) got it out of my way. I got in down on paper instead so…so it was not running through my brain (…) it was just the way it should be.
> L: well, for Kenny (…) I think (.) he has a very strong belief in his own optimism and it can carry him through (.) and I have (.) I have been very occupied with that. There is a cell biologist named Bruce Clipton who originally was a gene researcher and they are brought up with the idea that it's the genes, all about genes. Then he made some trails where it suddenly dawned on him that it's not about the genes, it's about the environment (.) Kenny and I have a strong belief that the environment around us and our relationship and love for each other and our self-respect – the fact that we both are working with our self-respect and our independence, that the environment is just as rewarding as to go somewhere [treatment abroad] and we are experiencing the effects of it.

A strong belief

Constructing a positive narrative about Lillian's condition was important for Kenny. However, being positive and having a strong belief in a positive outcome is a genuine characteristic for this couple's narrative identity. They construct a strong belief, but stress that it is not a religious belief, but a spiritual belief in something bigger. Lillian express it like this:

L: This entire metamorphosis our relationship has gone through has been amazing to experience. We are convinced that it will be a contributing factor to Kenny's recovery. Both now and what may come in the future. I don't…We have to talk a little bit about spirituality, because belief means a lot. Not like a church belief, but a belief in the fact that there is a creator and we are all highly beloved creatures and the day we recognize this, we will start to treat our self as beloved creatures (…) then a lot can change in our lives. In this sense, we are working on and thinking about a relationship to each other and a relation to the world. Being able to put worries and sorrows aside. In the beginning when I was discharged and started to deal with the fact that Kenny was ill (…) I was so scared. Then I had an extra session with the psychologist and she taught me some tricks and now I have worked with it spiritually and I know that I can put it aside, somebody else will take care of it. I have to concentrate on life, joy and being grateful.

C: Has this [spiritually] taken up a greater place after your injury?

L: Yes, a lot more.

C: But it has always been there?

Yes, always.

K: …but in another way in the beginning. We have stones and crystals and stuff like that which we have been working with and has previous read a lot of books on it. Everything has its own vibrations and frequencies.

A stronger and wiser husband

In the five-year follow-up interview, Lillian talks about the transition Kenny has gone through as a man. She describes herself as the dominating part of the relationship. In addition, she says that Kenny had a dominating mom, and now he has her. However, during her illness a transition has happened. Kenny took over and stepped into a new character:

L: So in many ways he is a much stronger and wiser man.

C: So this has been a gift to your relationship?

L: Very much.

K: mmm (confirming)

C: because even dominating woman thinks it is nice to have a man who …

L: yes

C: steps into character

L: yes

C: We just struggle to leave room for it.

L: Yes.

C: So …

L: and he has claimed that now

C: Yes, yes

L: and I am SO cautious to look after it. I am so grateful that he showed up.
C: Yes, amazing
Lillian and Kenny kiss each other.
L: yes, it is amazing. Beautiful, beautiful story.

We got a second chance

Kenny and Lillian have been together for more than 45 years. During the interviews with them, they are very affectionate and loving towards each other. They describe a growth and revitalization in their relationship because of what happened to them.

K: We got a second chance. We thought that we would only get that at reincarnation. You did not get that, right? (laughter) so we thought it was only then we would get another chance. But we got that now and we have grabbed that.
C: OK.
K: Every day is a gift and it should be fully enjoyed
K: We had a renaissance. We took it. We live here and now and we are feeling great.
L: Totally amazing.
C: Yes.
L: We love each other very much.
C: Yes.
K: Yes, yes.
L: I had a hard time saying it for some years before I got ill (…) I could not get the words out.
C: No.
L: Not that I did not [love him], but our relationship was a bit worn out and complicated.
C: Yes, yes
L: Now, I tell him 7 days a week. You need to say it while we have each other (…)
C: Yes.
L: For me it is a conscious mindset (.) like a muscle that needs to be trained like any other muscle.
C: Yes, OK.
L: It is a brain capacity that needs to be trained like any other brain capacity. If you focus on it.

Both their illnesses became the starting point of a new beginning in their relationship. After more than 45 years, the relationship was worn out and complicated. Yet, again we see how spirituality becomes a mediator for finding ease with a situation. They had already discussed their relationship, and talked about a new beginning, but only after reincarnation. However, a transformation happened after their illness. Their love and relationship were revitalized.

Discussion

The chapter has explored "post-traumatic growth" (PTG) in families affected by an ABI. Through a case study, this chapter has illustrated how spirituality, acceptance, and committed actions in regards to finding new meaning and choosing a positive mindset can help couples to PTG after an ABI. Furthermore, it revealed how illness can reconstruct and change positions in a relationship in a positive way and recreate a strong bond as a couple. Therefore, a traumatic event can be the starting point of a new beginning including personal and relational growth.

Lillian and Kenny's narratives about having a strong will and choosing a positive mindset resonate with the saying "your mind can move mountains". Committed actions and choosing a positive mindset can be referred to as training a positive muscle that involves an active choice to see possibilities and prioritizing resources to committed action. Positive thinking does not necessarily mean avoiding or ignoring bad things. It involves making the most of the potential bad situation, and viewing yourself and your abilities in a positive light. Accepting what is not yet changeable is a part of taking committed action on what can be changed. In that sense, committed action gives the possibilities of PTG.

Our study also gave insight into how the same situation can be perceived and narrated quite differently from a professional's perspective and a first-person ABI survivor's perspective or relative's perspective. There are various examples of professionals' interpretations becoming the official story while the stories, the voices, and the experiences of the couple are changed or silenced. This concerns questions such as: who gets to define what is progress? Whose directives are followed and whose are silenced? Kenny kept and narrated a positive mindset in emails to family and friends and in this way also kept hoping for a positive outcome despite doctors' prognosis. When clients or relatives are encouraged to keep their hopes realistic, that is, limited to what their official prognosis predicts, they have to live through the distress of abandoning previous life ideals and aspirations in the sense of Frank and Frank (1991). Barnard (1995) has focused on the "dynamics of hoping" in the context of chronic illness, emphasizing that patients are set to live in the tension of a particularly troubling boundary situation; that is, "the boundary between old formulations of the self and new formulations not yet born" (p. 50). Narratives are suggested to perform a vital role in constructing possibilities that enable people to engage with different modalities of hope.

Central for this case study is how Lillian and Kenny cope with the situation as a unit. Kenny and Lillian are in a consolidated marriage and, thus, have a long experience of developing coping abilities as a couple. In the last 20 years a new attention towards interpersonal aspects of coping has emerged (Revenson et al., 2005; Kayser & Scott, 2008; Iafrate & Donato, 2012; Regan et al., 2015; Traa, De Vries, Bodenmann, & Den Oudsten, 2015). Therefore, couples' coping has started to be conceptualized no longer referring to the separate perspectives of the two partners, but as a dyadic process involving their mutual influence (Bodenmann, 1997). Dyadic coping is conceptualized as a process shaped by the individual's close relationships (Bodenmann, 2005; Revenson et al., 2005). It is described as "the interplay between the stress signals of one partner and the coping reactions of the other, a genuine act of shared coping" (Revenson et al., 2005, p. 4). Through a series of interactions, dyadic coping contributes to a sense of we-ness and promotes the conjoint creation of strategies to respond to the stressful event (Revenson, 1994; Bodenmann, 1997; Scott, Halford, & Ward, 2004; Kayser, Watson, & Andrade, 2007).

Longitudinal studies have confirmed that dyadic coping represents a protective factor for the couple's relationship, with better relational outcomes and a reduced risk of being divorced registered among dyads reporting common coping (Bodenmann & Cina, 2005; Bodenmann, Pihet, & Kayser, 2006). However, a significant gap in the literature is the understanding of how the life stage of couples may influence their dyadic coping and the accompanying quality of life. Previous research indicates that younger couples are more vulnerable to distress, experience poorer quality of life, and appear to be at risk for negative adjustment to the stress of the illness because of four reasons. First, it has been documented that coping abilities increase with age, with older individuals presenting better emotion regulation and more effective collaborative coping skills (i.e. Folkman, Lazarus, Pimley, & Novacek, 1987; Revenson, 2003; Helgeson, Snyder, & Seltman, 2004; Revenson & Pranikoff, 2005). Second, contextual and generational factors may impact younger couples' vulnerabilities, as younger generations report higher levels of stress, often associated with financial insecurity and unhealthy lifestyles, when compared with previous generations (American Psychological Association, 2015). Third, while there is little disagreement that marital satisfaction decreases with time (Bradbury & Karney, 2014), the literature about close relationships has provided over the last decades evidence of relational and psychological difficulties for newlyweds and younger families (Carstensen, Fung, & Charles, 2003; Carstensen et al., 2011; Woszidlo & Segrin, 2013; Bradbury & Karney, 2014).

While initial studies showed that older couples perform consistently better than younger ones (Revenson, 2003; Revenson & Pranikoff, 2005; Berg & Upchurch, 2007; Hoppmann, Coats, & Blanchard-Fields, 2008), others have highlighted stereotypical similarity in younger couples (Iafrate & Donato, 2012). The authors concluded that younger partners appear to experience a heightened perceived idealization of the relationship. A recent study analysed stress, dyadic coping, and partners' well-being in three age cohorts (Cohort 1: 20–35 years old; Cohort 2: 40–55 years old; Cohort 3: 65–80 years old). Among the younger cohort, women's well-being was affected by stress and negative supportive behaviours, while males' quality of life was mostly influenced by individual coping and contextual factors (Vedes, Nussbeck, & Bodenmann, 2015). Among middle-aged couples, the well-being of both partners was influenced by stress and dyadic coping. While investigators found an actor effect for female partners, the well-being of male partners appeared to be more dependent on the dyadic coping of the wife. These differences disappeared in the late-adulthood group. It is therefore possible to conclude that the relationship among stress, dyadic coping, and well-being changes across the life course experience.

Conclusion

Traditionally, research has focused on the negative consequences of ABI. However, the fact that a substantial proportion of people with ABI do not develop psychological distress means that positive and protective mechanisms are also worthy of consideration. Over the decade there has been an increase in people subscribing to the idea that positive growth may be possible after ABI, particularly when changes occur in relation to a person's sense of meaning, purpose, heightened spirituality, and enhanced relationships after brain injury.

In our case study, we found that dyadic coping contributes to a sense of weness and promotes the conjoint creation of strategies to respond to the stressful event caused by illness and create post-traumatic growth. Such strategies can be a choosing a positive mindset, spirituality, and creating positive illness narratives.

The present chapter concludes that research in ABI would be enhanced by incorporation of the relatively new concept of "post-traumatic growth", not least because it offers a psychologically grounded entrée into the area of spirituality in ABI survivors and partners.

References

Affleck, G., Tennen, H., Croog, S., & Levine, S. (1987). Causal attribution, perceived benefits and morbidity after a heart attack: An 8-year study. *Journal of Consulting and Clinical Psychology*, 55, 29–35.

Anderson, M., Parmenter, T., & Mok, M. (2002). The relationship between neurobehavioural problems of severe traumatic brain injury (TBI), family functioning and the psychological well-being of the spouse/caregiver: Path model analysis. *Brain Injury*, 16, 743–757. doi:10.1080/02699050210128906.

Bamberg, M. (2003). Positioning with Davie Hogan: Stories, tellings, and identities. In C. Daiute and C. Lightfoot (Eds.), *Narrative analysis: Studying the development of individuals in society* (pp. 135–157). London: Sage.

Bamberg, M. (2011). Who am I? Narration and its contribution to self and identity. *Theory & Psychology*, 21(1), 3–24.

Bamberg, M. & Georgakopoulou, A. (2008). Small stories as a new perspective in narrative and identity analysis. *Text & Talk: An Interdisciplinary Journal of Language, Discourse & Communication Studies*, 28(3), 377–396.

Bamberg, M., De Fina, A., & Schiffrin, D. (2011). Discourse and identity construction. In S.J. Schwartz, V.L. Vignoles, & K. Luyckx (Eds.), *Handbook of identity theory and research* (pp. 1–23). New York: Springer.

Barnard, D. (1995). Chronic illness and the dynamics of hoping. In S.K. Toombs, D. Barnard, & R.A. Carson (Eds.), *Chronic illness: From experience to policy* (pp. 38–57). Bloomington: Indiana University Press.

Berg, C.A. & Upchurch, R. (2007). A developmental-contextual model of couples coping with chronic illness across the adult life span. *Psychological Bulletin*, 133(6), 920–954. doi:10.1037/0033-2909.133.6.920.

Bodenmann, G. (1997). Dyadic coping: A systemic-transactional view of stress and coping among couples: Theory and empirical findings. *European Review of Applied Psychology*, 47, 137–140.

Bodenmann, G. (2005). Dyadic coping and its significance for marital functioning. In T.A. Revenson, K. Kayser, & G. Bodenmann (Eds.), *Couples coping with stress: Emerging perspectives on dyadic coping* (pp. 33–49). Washington, DC: American Psychological Association.

Bodenmann, G. & Cina, A. (2005). Stress and coping among stable-satisfied, stable-distressed and separated/divorced Swiss couples: A 5-years prospective longitudinal study. *Journal of Divorce & Remarriage*, 44, 71–89. doi:10.1300/J087v44n01_04.

Bodenmann, G., Pihet, S., & Kayser, K. (2006). The relationship between dyadic coping and marital quality: A 2-year longitudinal study. *Journal of Family Psychology*, 20, 485–493. doi:10.1037/0893-3200.20.3.485.

Bombardier, C.H., Fann, J.R., Temkin, N.R., Esselman, P.C., Barber, J., & Dikmen, S. S. (2010). Rates of major depressive disorder and clinical outcomes following traumatic brain injury. *Journal of the American Medical Association*, 303(19),1938–1945. doi:10.1001/jama.2010.599.

Bowen, C., Yeates, G., & Palmer, S. (2010). *A relational approach to rehabilitation: Thinking about relationships after brain injury*. London: Karnac Books.

Bower, J.E., Moskowitz, J.T., & Epel, E. (2009). Is benefit finding good for your health? Pathways linking positive life changes after stress and physical health outcomes. *Current Directions in Psychological Science*, 18(6), 337–341.

Bower, J.E., Kemeny, M.E., Taylor, S.E., & Fahey, J.L. (1998). Cognitive processing, discovery of meaning, CD4 decline, and AIDS related mortality among bereaved HIV-seropositive men. *Journal of Consulting and Clinical Psychology*, 66, 979–986.

Bradbury, T.N., & Karney, B.R. (2014). *Intimate relationships*. New York: W.W. Norton and Company.

Brain Injury Association of Queensland. (2010). *Get the facts: Acquired brain injury fact sheets* [*Fact sheet*]. Retrieved from: www.synapse.org/get-the-facts.aspx.

Braun, V. & Clarke, V. (2006). Using thematic analysis in psychology. *Qualitative Research in Psychology*, 3(2), 77–101.

Brooks, D.N. (1991). The head-injured family. *Journal of Clinical Experimental Neuropsychology*, 13(1), 155–188.

Carnes, S.L. & Quinn, W.H. (2005). Family adaptation to brain injury: Coping and psychological distress. *Families, Systems, & Health*, 23, 186–203. doi:10.1037/1091-7527.23.2.186.

Carstensen, L.L., Fung, H., & Charles, S. (2003). Socioemotional selectivity theory and the regulation of emotion in the second half of life. *Motivation and Emotion*, 27, 103–123. doi:10.1023/A:1024569803230.

Carstensen, L.L., Turan, B., Scheibe, S., Ram, N., Ersner-Hershfield, H., Samanez-Larkin, G. R., et al. (2011). Emotional experience improves with age: Evidence based on over 10 years of experience sampling. *Psychology and Aging*, 26, 21–33. doi:10.1037/a0021285.

Cassidy, T. (2012). Benefit finding through caring: The cancer caregiver experience. *Psychology & Health*, 28(3), 250–266. doi:10.1080/08870446.2012.717623.

Cassidy, T., Giles, M., & McLaughlin, M. (2013). Benefit finding and resilience in child caregivers. *British Journal of Health Psychology*, 19(3), 606–618. doi:10.1111/bjhp.12059.

Davies, B., & Harré, R. (1990). Positioning: The discursive production of selves. *Journal for the Theory of Social Behavior*, 20(1), 43–63.

De Fina, A., Schiffrin, D., & Bamberg, M. (2006). Introduction. In A. De Fina, D. Schiffrin, & M. Bamberg (Eds.), *Discourse and identity* (pp. 1–23). Cambridge: Cambridge University Press.

Evans, J.J. (2011). Positive psychology and brain injury rehabilitation. *Brain Impairment*, 12, 117–127. doi:10.1375/brim.12.2.117.

Folkman, S., Lazarus, R.S., Pimley, S., & Novacek, J. (1987). Age differences in stress and coping processes. *Psychology and Aging*, 2, 171–184. doi:10.1037/0882-7974.2.2.171.

Frank, J.D. & Frank, J.A. (1991). *Persuasion and healing: A comparative study of psychotherapy* (3rd Edition). Baltimore: Johns Hopkins University Press.

Frankl, V. (1963). *Man's search for meaning*. New York: Washington SquarePress.

Gill, C., Sander, A., Robins, N., Mazzei, D., & Struchen, M. (2011). Exploring experiences of intimacy from the viewpoint of individuals with traumatic brain injury and their partners. *The Journal of Head Trauma Rehabilitation*, 26, 56–68. doi:10.1097/HTR.0b013e3182048ee9.

Glintborg, C. (2015). Grib mennesket. En konceptuel og empirisk undersøgelse af koordineret rehabilitering: objektivt bio-psyko-socialt udbytte for voksne med erhvervet hjerneskade samt klienters og pårørendes oplevelse af rehabiliteringen med og uden kommunal koordination. Ph.D.-afhandling. Det Humanistiske Fakultet, Aalborg Universitets Forlag. www.hcci.aau.dk/digitalAssets/129/129472_chalotte_glintborg_phd-afhandling.pdf.

Glintborg, C. (2019). *Identity reconstruction after brain injury: Personal and family identity*. New York: Routledge.

Glintborg, C. & Hansen, T. (2016). Bio-psycho-social effects of a coordinated neurorehabilitation programme: A naturalistic mixed methods study. *NeuroRehabilitation*, 38, 99–113. doi:10.3233/NRE-161301.

Glintborg, C. & Hansen, T.G.B. (in press). Psychosocial sequelae after acquired brain injury: a 5-year follow-up study.

Hackett, M.L. & Anderson, C.S. (2005). Predictors of depression after stroke: A systematic review of observational studies. *Stroke*, 36, 2296–2301.

Helgeson, V.S., Reynolds, K.A., & Tomich, P.L. (2006). A meta-analytic review of benefit finding and growth. *Journal of Consulting and Clinical Psychology*, 74(5), 797–816.

Helgeson, V.S., Snyder, P., & Seltman, H. (2004). Psychological and physical adjustment to breast cancer over 4 years: Identifying distinct trajectories of change. *Health Psychology*, 23, 3–15. doi:10.1037/0278-6133.23.1.3.

Hoppmann, C.A., Coats, A.H., & Blanchard-Fields, F. (2008). Goals and everyday problem solving: Examining the link between age-related goals and problem-solving strategy use. neuropsychology, development, and cognition. *Cognitive Neuropsychology*, 15, 401–423. doi:10.1080/13825580701533777.

Iafrate, R. & Donato, S. (2012). Coping in a relational context: The case of dyadic coping. In B. Molinelli & V. Grimaldo (Eds.), *Handbook of the psychology of coping: New research* (pp. 11–132). Hauppauge: Nova Science Publishers.

Janoff-Bulman, R. (1992). *Shattered assumptions: Towards a new psychology of trauma*. New York: The Free Press.

Kayser, K. & Scott, J.L. (2008). *Helping couples cope with women's cancers: An evidence-based approach for practitioners*. New York: Springer.

Kayser, K., Watson, E., & Andrade, J.T. (2007). Cancer as a we-disease: Examining the process of coping from a relational perspective. *Families, Systems, & Health*, 25, 404–418. doi:10.1037/1091-7527.25.4.404.
Kolakowsky-Hayner, S.A., Miner, K.D., & Kreutzer, J.S. (2001). Long-term life quality and family needs after traumatic brain injury. *The Journal of Head Trauma Rehabilitation*, 16, 374–385. doi:10.1097/00001199-200108000-00007.
Kreutzer, J.S., Gervasio, A.H., & Camplair, P.S. (1994). Primary caregivers' psychological status and family functioning after traumatic brain injury. *Brain Injury*, 8, 197–210. doi:10.3109/02699059409150973.
Kreutzer, J.S., Marwitz, J.H., Hsu, N., Williams, K., & Riddick, A. (2007). Marital stability after brain injury: An investigation and analysis. *NeuroRehabilitation*, 22 (1), 53–59.
Lazarus, R.S. & Folkman, S. (1984). *Stress, appraisal and coping*. New York: Springer.
Lezak, M.D. (1986). Psychological implications of traumatic brain damage for the patient's family. *Rehabilitation Psychology*, 31, 241–250. doi:10.1037/h0091551.
Lezak, M.D. (1988). Brain damage is a family affair. *Journal of Clinical and Experimental Neuropsychology*, 10, 111–123. doi:10.1080/01688638808405098.
Linley, P.A. & Joseph, S. (Eds.) (2004). *Positive psychology in practice*. Hoboken: John Wiley & Sons.
McAdams, D.P. (1993). *The stories we live by: Personal myths and the making of the self*. New York: William Morrow & Co.
McGrath, J., & King, N. (2004). Acquired brain injury. In J. Bennett-Levy, G. Butler, M. Fennell, A. Hackman, M. Mueller, & D. Westbrook (Eds.), *The Oxford guide to behavioural experiments* (pp. 331–350). Oxford: Oxford University Press.
McGregor, B.A. & Antoni, M.H. (2009). Psychological intervention and health outcomes among women treated for breast cancer: A review of stress pathways and biological mediators. *Brain Behavior and Immunity*, 23, 159–166.
McIntosh, D. (1995). Religion-as-schema with implications for the relation between religion and coping. *International Journal for the Psychology of Religion*, 5, 1–16.
McMillen, J.C., & Fisher, R.H. (1998). The perceived benefit scales: Measuring perceived positive life changes after negative events. *Social Work Research*, 22, 173–186.
Masel, B. & DeWitt, D.S. (2010). Traumatic brain injury: A disease process, not an event. *Journal of Neurotrauma*, 27, 1529–1540. doi:10.1089/neu.2010.1358.
Mauss-Clum, N. & Ryan, M. (1981). Brain injury and the family. *Journal of Neuroscience Nursing*, 13, 165–169.
Miller, W. & C'de Baca, J. (2001). *Quantum change: When epiphanies and sudden insights transform ordinary lives*. New York: Guilford.
Nabors, N., Seacat, J., & Rosenthal, M. (2002). Predictors of caregiver burden following traumatic brain injury. *Brain Injury*, 16, 1039–1050. doi:10.1080/02699050210155285.
Nochi, M. (2000). Reconstructing self-narratives in coping with traumatic brain injury. *Social Science & Medicine*, 51(12), 1795–1804. doi:10.1016/S0277-9536(00)00111-8.
Pargament, K.I. (1997). *The psychology of religion and coping: Theory, research, practice*. New York: Guilford Press.
Potter, J. & Wetherell, M. (1987). *Discourse and social psychology: Beyond attitudes and behaviour*. London: Sage.
Regan, T.W., Lambert, S.D., Kelly, B., Falconier, M., Kissane, D., & Levesque, J.V. (2015). Couples coping with cancer: Exploration of theoretical frameworks from dyadic studies. *Psychooncology*, 24, 1605–1617. doi:10.1002/pon.3854.

Revenson, T.A. (1994). Social support and marital coping with chronic illness. *Annals of Behavioral Medicine*, 16, 122–130.
Revenson, T.A. (2003). Scenes from a marriage: Examining support and marital coping with chronic illness. In J. Suls & K. Wallston (Eds.), *Social psychological foundations of health and illness* (pp. 530–559). Oxford: Blackwell.
Revenson, T.A. & Pranikoff, J.R. (2005). A contextual approach to treatment decision making among breast cancer survivors. *Health Psychology*, 24, S93–S98. doi:10.1037/0278-6133.24.4.S93.
Revenson, T.A., Kayser, K., & Bodenmann, G. (2005). *Emerging perspectives on couples' coping with stress*. Washington, DC: American Psychological Association.
Scott, J.L., Halford, W.K., & Ward, B.G. (2004). United we stand? The effects of a couple-coping intervention on adjustment to early stage breast or gynaecological cancer. *The Journal of Consulting and Clinical Psychology*, 72, 1122–1135. doi:10.1037/0022-006X.72.6.1122.
Seel, R.T., Macciocchi, S., & Kreutzer, J.S. (2010). Clinical considerations for the diagnosis of major depression after moderate to severe TBI. *The Journal of Head Trauma Rehabilitation*, 25, 99–112. doi:10.1097/HTR.0b013e3181ce3966.
Tedeschi, R.G. & Calhoun, L.G. (1995). *Trauma & transformation: Growing in the aftermath of suffering*. Sage.
Tedeschi, R.G. & Calhoun, L.G. (2004). The posttraumatic growth inventory: Measuring the positive legacy of trauma. *Journal of Traumatic Stress*, 9, 455–471.
Tennen, H. & Affleck, G. (2002). Benefit-finding and benefit-reminding. In C.R. Snyder & S.J. Lopez (Eds.), *The handbook of positive psychology* (pp. 279–304). New York: Oxford University Press.
Tomich, P.L. & Helgeson, V.S. (2004). Is finding something good in the bad always good? Benefit finding among women with breast cancer. *Health Psychology*, 23, 16–23.
Traa, M.J., De Vries, J., Bodenmann, G., & Den Oudsten, B.L. (2015). Dyadic coping and relationship functioning in couples coping with cancer: A systematic review. *British Journal of Health Psychology*, 20, 85–114. doi:10.1111/bjhp.12094.
Ullman, C. (1982). Cognitive and emotional antecedents of religious conversion. *Journal of Personality & Social Psychology*, 43, 183–192.
Vedes, A., Nussbeck, F., & Bodenmann, G. (2015). A life cycle perspective on stress, dyadic coping and couples' well-being. Paper presented at the 9th Workshopkongress für Klinische Psychologie und Psychoterapie/33. Symposim der Fachgruppe Klinische Psychologie und Psychotherapie der DGPs (Dresden).
Woszidlo, A. & Segrin, C. (2013). Negative affectivity and educational attainment as predictors of newlyweds' problem solving communication and marital quality. *The Journal of Psychology*, 147, 49–73. doi:10.1080/00223980.2012.674069.
Zasler, N.D., Katz, D.I., Zafonte, R.D., Arciniegas, D.B., Bullock, M.R., & Kreutzer, J.S. (Eds.) (2012). *Brain injury medicine: Principles and practice* (2nd Edition). New York: Demos Medical.

5 Narrative identity and dementia

The problem of living with fewer available resources

Lars-Christer Hydén and Mattias Forsblad

Introduction

A growing number of researchers have argued that both identity and self are narrative: a person's identity develops and changes through a constant narrative elaboration and revision. Disorders like Alzheimer's disease (AD) – as well as many other brain disorders – challenge the idea of a connection between human identity and stories. The reason for this is that persons living with dementia are challenged in the use of those cognitive and linguistic resources needed to tell and understand stories. Thus, persons with dementia tend to tell autobiographical stories that often deviate from cultural narrative norms and expectations.

Still, storytelling is a relevant activity for the person with dementia at all the different stages of the disease process for the simple reason that both the person with dementia and other family members have much of their identity invested in everyday stories, and they all continue to tell stories even when the person with dementia has severe problems with telling the stories. Thus, being able to take part in storytelling implies being able to sustain relations and identities.

In dementia the pathological brain processes change the functional systems of the brain and thus the resources central in the construction of narrative identities (episodic memory for instance) become less available for the person living with dementia as the disorder progresses. As a consequence, the patterns of engagement of the person with dementia in storytelling activities will change over time. Some persons with dementia can tell autobiographical stories on their own, while others can do it with support, especially from someone that has known them for a longer period, while others at a later stage of dementia are extremely challenged in making contributions to autobiographical storytelling.

Central to the narrative challenges for people living with dementia is the decreasing resources available for constructing, telling, and understanding autobiographical stories. In this chapter we will focus on and discuss how both persons living with dementia as well as other participants can compensate the loss of resources. We will do this by discussing the concept of identity in relation to narrative and storytelling. Our main argument will be around the idea that the changes in the brain brought about by the various dementia disorders translate into a loss of resources that can compensated for through the use of alternative resources. These can be found among the individual's own remaining cognitive resources, as well as in other participants and as external cultural resources.

Autobiographical stories and identity

For many researchers, clinicians, and writers, identity is constituted by or consists of narratives. It is by telling stories about ourselves and our lives that we show who and what we are. Through the creation, elaboration, and revision of autobiographical narratives we both develop and possess an identity and a sense of ourselves as persons – a sense of self (Brockmeier & Carbaugh, 2001; Brockmeier, 2015; Bruner, 2001).

Narratives can be used in several ways in order to tell or show something about who the teller is and what kind of person he or she is – or has been. One obvious possibility inherent in narratives is to connect the past with the present by telling stories about how events in the past have led to the situation at the time of telling the story (Bamberg, 2011). The autobiographical story can stress the sameness of the person by stressing continuity in life over time (McAdams, 2006). Another possibility is to point to a fundamental disruption and change in life, through events that have been halting or changing the course of the life process, and thus to tell a story including turning points (McAdams, Josselson, & Lieblich, 2001). In focusing on either continuity or change it is primarily the discursive organization of the autobiographical narrative that is in focus, especially the narrative's temporal and referential aspects.

Autobiographical stories and storytelling have at least three aspects of relevance in this context. One, from a *cognitive* perspective the central aspect of an autobiographical story is the temporal and causal connection of two or more events into a coherent whole (Chafe, 1994; Labov, 1972). That is, at the heart of an autobiographical story is the effort to create meaning by connecting events together, and maintain that events not just follow on from each other temporally but are causally connected: one event causes or leads to the other event. This aspect of storytelling is dependent on various memory systems: from episodic and semantic memory system in order to identify relevant events, to working memory and planning (Mar, 2004). Two, from a *linguistic* point of view, most stories are discursive constructions that go beyond the simple utterance (or sentence) and this implies connecting a number of clauses, main as well as sub-clauses, into a longer discourse (Genette, 1980). This puts strain on both basic and more advanced linguistic resources as well as memory systems, especially working memory (Mar, 2004). Three, from an *interactional* perspective, it can be noted that although autobiographical stories are about one individual (the teller), most stories of this type are told in conversations. Other people may share knowledge and experiences from the events the teller refers to and may want to revise and negotiate the story. Autobiographical stories told in conversational settings are thus often joint constructions rather than individual expressions (Ochs & Capps, 2001). That is, although a teller may be considered to be the author and main protagonist of the story, other participants may make new contributions to the story or question parts of it.

Each of these three aspects of autobiographical stories and storytelling also represent the major areas of challenges and opportunities for people living with dementia, as will be discussed in the following.

Stories, identities and dementia

Dementia is an umbrella term for a number of diseases that affect the brain's ability to function cognitively and linguistically. Different areas and sub-systems in the brain are affected by different types of dementia. In AD it is primarily the various memory systems that are affected at first, in particular episodic memory as well as semantic and working memory. Vascular dementia may also affect memory systems, while frontotemporal dementia often affects the social control of behaviour (Lezak, Howieson, Bigler, & Tranel, 2012). Some forms of AD and frontotemporal dementias primarily affects those parts of the brain involved in language production and understanding (semantic dementia, primary progressive aphasia) (Wilson et al., 2010).

As a result of the impairments to areas and parts of the brain involved in cognition and language, the person living with dementia will be communicatively challenged. Impairments to the brain imply that functions that normally serve as *resources* or building blocks for constructing for instance autobiographical stories, are no longer available. Resources can for instance consist of vocabulary (the words that are available), prosody (available prosodic tunes), gestures (mimic, pointing, etc.) as well as cognitive content like remembered events and facts (various memory systems) (Perkins, 2007; Goodwin, 2017). The person living with dementia might have fewer available words and names as well as fewer storylines to choose from in telling an autobiographical story (see Örulv & Hydén, 2006). The impairments to the brain caused by for instance the neurodegenerative processes are from an interactional perspective translated into a shrinking of the number of available resources. Having fewer available resources implies that the functional systems consisting of many different resources coordinated to produce a contribution to an ongoing activity, will be affected (Perkins, 2007). That is, in order to tell a story both different cognitive (various kinds of memories) and linguistic resources (words, syntactic constructions) must be used and coordinated into what has been called functional systems (or neural networks) (Luria, 1973).

As a consequence, stories told by persons with dementia are often perceived as *broken stories* because they are often fragmented, jumbled, and repetitive, and lack temporal and thematic coherence (Hydén & Brockmeier, 2008). Further, storytellers as well as listeners risk becoming *entangled* in these broken stories as beginnings and endings are twisted together, interwoven with repetitions of the same event, resulting in shared states of narrative perplexity (Hydén, 2018).

Although stories told by persons living with dementia can be broken, the telling of autobiographical stories is still used to perform and claim identity (Bitenc, 2018; Hydén, 2018). Over time, as the dementia disorder progresses, there will be changes in how the person living with dementia participates in storytelling events. In the beginning, the person can still take part as an active teller, presenting autobiographical stories although with some support in particular concerning repair work (Hydén, 2011). As the disorder progresses through the middle phase and eventually the final stage, the voice of the person with dementia becomes weaker and the supportive tellings of relatives or others may start to function as vicarious voices. At first by supplementing story elements, later on by substituting both the actual voice and the authorship of the story from the person living with dementia (Hydén, 2008, 2018).

Thus, although the person with dementia faces increasing challenges, for quite a long time it is still possible to voice autobiographical stories. One of the main challenges for the person with dementia voicing his or her own story is how to deal with and compensate for the fact that fewer cognitive and linguistic resources are available. Most persons living with dementia develop both individual compensatory strategies as well as collaborative adaptive strategies involving others (Hydén, 2018). Some of the compensatory strategies focus on what the individual can do to use alternative resources or use actually available resources in new ways. Many of these strategies have to do with how to deal with memory and linguistic resources. Other strategies have to do with how the resources of other persons can be elicited and used in order to produce an autobiographical story, for instance getting someone else to provide a name or a memory of an event.

We argue that some insights about coping with fewer available resources can be gained if we combine the interest for narrative identity and autobiographical storytelling with interactive theories about cognition (see, for instance, Hutchins, 1995; Hollan, Hutchins, & Kirsh, 2000). The focus of these theoretical perspectives is on how people accomplish tasks together in joint activities. In doing things together the participants must coordinate their actions, including their attentional, cognitive, and linguistic resources, and the participants need to focus their senses and cognition on the shared environment. As a consequence of this it makes sense to talk about the participants and their bodily, cognitive, and linguistic activity as part of a common system rather than as individual actions and states not related to the ongoing joint activity. In doing things together, the participants are also committed to be relevant and supportive (Bratman, 1992; Gilbert, 1990).

In the following we would like to focus on three types of adaptive strategies in order to use available resources: (1) individual cognitive resources; (2) social resources, that is, the resources of other people; and (3) cultural resources, in particular in using artefacts. We are in particular interested in how these resources can be used to meet and overcome the challenges the dementia disorder presents; that is, the compensatory possibilities inherent in interactional storytelling.

Individual cognitive and linguistic resources for narrative identity

Historically, the notion of a close connection between memories and identity has been at the centre of much of the writings about personal identity. Identity is assumed to be based on recollection of previous personal memories. In theories about narrative identity, it is assumed that the stories are based on remembered events that are turned into stories.

In particular AD challenges this connection between identity and memory as persons living with AD are challenged in both "creating" and "recalling" memories and could hence not have or sustain an identity. As a result, persons with AD will "lose" their identity as consequence of "losing" autobiographical memories.

Interestingly, much of the current empirically based literature on dementia and identity argue against the assumption that failing memory leads to a loss of self for people with dementia (for a review, see Hydén, 2020). One reason for this might be that autobiographical storytelling from a neuro-scientific perspective entails neural networks or functional systems that draw on and are dependent on a number of other networks (lower functions), i.e. episodic and semantic memory, working memory, linguistic constructions, etc. It is by being connected and working together that these neural networks can serve their function in storytelling events. When basic functions in this extended network are not available it is possible for the brain to undergo a re-organization of the involved processes rather than a loss. Thus, it would be possible for the individual to make use of other available resources in the brain.

In a study, Strikwerda-Brown, Grilli, Andrews-Hanna, and Irish (2019) made a comparison between AD, semantic dementia (SD), and the behavioural variant of frontotemporal dementia (bvFTD) and argued that persons can use a number of different compensatory strategies based on the continuity of self across these diseases. Persons with AD are for instance noted to lose the subjective self-continuity in numerous ways but can still be able to know that, and how, events took place; especially from the more distant past that rely more on semantic memory resources. Grounding the self in the more distant past increases the likelihood of putting oneself in the present and "who I was" can therefore become "who I am" (Strikwerda-Brown et al., 2019).

Patients with SD, on the other hand, are noted to recollect recent events while episodes from the longer past lack details that can be adhered to a loss of semantic memory resources. Strikwerda-Brown and colleagues (2019) therefore hypothesize that people with SD rely more on recent events to define the self. Note that recent events can be a story from the remote past told in the present through for instance co-constructed storytelling, and therefore SD patients can potentially retain a higher level of functioning than AD patients.

People with bvFTD are also noted to experience a loss of subjective self-continuity but, unlike AD patients, this happens through a breakdown of social functioning. The later breakdown of episodic and semantic memory functioning further damages the social functioning. Persons with AD and SD have an inbuilt compensatory mechanism for a narrative self across what

Strikwerda-Brown et al. (2019) name the episodic and semantic continuum. The continuum is roughly specified involving four types of utterances: specific events, general events, personal semantics, and general semantics.

A case study of two women, one with dementia, in an American rural working-class setting, also concluded that identity is not lost in people with dementia and gave examples of narratives the person with dementia returns to from youth and old age (Shenk, Davis, Peacock, & Moore, 2002). Although the stories told by the woman demanded co-construction across occasions the themes of the narratives were consistent with stories from a gender-based working class; where rural American cultural values are dominant and which included closeness of family, hard work, ties to the land, and religious faith. Again, this points towards people with dementia being able to use other resources to claim identities. In this case the utterances can perhaps be understood as drawing from general and personal semantics such as knowledge and values of the past that allow for fragmented, but nevertheless functional, narratives.

Another study by Eustache et al. (2013) confirms part of the compensatory mechanism across the episodic–semantic continuum by investigating the preservation of identity among 16 patients with AD (mild to severe) and 16 controls across two sets of testing a fortnight in between. In one part of the study participants were asked to finish ten so-called "I am" statements which perhaps can be understood as a very structured and simplistic form of a narrative identity. Answers were categorized as belonging to one of the following categories: idiocentric (e.g. I am an enthusiastic person), small group (e.g. I am a grandfather), large group (e.g. I am a pensioner), allocentric (e.g. I am a sociable person). Seven more concrete subcategories to these and emotional valence of utterances were also used.

Results show that four of the participants with AD said things that could not be correct. Six explicitly said things that referred to their lack of self-knowledge and overall AD patients reported fewer statements. However, there were no difference between persons with AD and controls in terms of response distribution across the categories and subcategories. This suggest that identity for persons with AD do not necessarily lose the expressed complexity involved in the higher cognitive function of identity despite that sub-identity functions are not working as they used to.

A fortnight later the above procedure was repeated to investigate the stability of the findings and no differences in terms of performance and distribution was found for the AD patients or controls. But interestingly there was a qualitative difference between the groups for the statements that were repetitions from previous testing (24.5% for AD and 20.3% for controls). AD participants made almost only verbatim repetitions while the controls made only rephrased repetitions. A tendency was that verbatim repetitions were more common among the participants with severe AD. Authors suggest that a core identity remains as a rigid resource for telling someone who you are despite being in advanced stages of AD. In other words, persons with AD are more likely to rely on semantic resources of who they are, and a hypothesis is therefore that the likelihood of doing so increases along the stages of the disease.

A review of 33 empirical studies on self in dementia conducted by Caddell and Clare (2010) confirms the above studies and finds that all studies find some persistence of self and identity in all stages of dementia diseases. They further note that studies with a qualitative approach tend to focus on the verbal aspects and to a lesser extent on the non-verbal. The quantitative approaches on the other hand are more likely to focus on short forms of utterances such as fact-questions, self-recognition, and, as mentioned above, "I am" statements that display minimalistic forms of narrative identity.

In conclusion, although the notion that memory and identity are closely connected, it seems to have a questionable empirical ground. Loss of memory (in particular episodic memory and autobiographical memory) do not automatically lead to a loss of identity. Rather, it seems that people living with dementia and whose brains are affected by the pathological processes involved in the specific types of dementia, can use a number of alternative resources for creating and sustaining a personal identity. Thus, it seems that identity is an opportunistic construction using those resources in the brain that are available as well as other types of, for instance cultural, resources.

Using other people: distributed memories and scaffolding

While some compensatory strategies might be about using the individual's remaining resources in new and functional ways, some resources can be found outside the individual. Memories of events, facts, and words might be something other participants have access to and the individual living with dementia can make use of these resources in order to tell an autobiographical story. Often couples, families, and friends have knowledge of each other's stories and share personal knowledge of each other because they have known each other for a long time; often they also have shared experiences. That is, they share a common ground. In residential care settings one way to expand the common ground between professional carers and persons with dementia is to systematically make use of life story work. That is, the person with dementia and relatives share the individual's life stories with staff and hence help the staff to "know" the person with dementia by suggesting an interpretative context for that individual, making it easier to interact with the person (McKeown, Clarke, & Repper, 2006; Surr, 2006).

As the person living with dementia become increasingly restricted in terms of available resources, for instance memories, relatives or staff can take over the autobiographical memories of the individual and thus become the "bearer" of these memories. When other persons around the person with dementia become holders of memories, the person with dementia can use these other persons as potential resources for "remembering" both events and personal knowledge. The person living with dementia can accomplish this by, for instance, requesting information from the healthy spouse and adding this to what he or she already "knows" and thus present an identity; or by letting other persons tell personal identity stories but claim ownership and responsibility of the stories and use them for presenting an identity (see Goodwin, 2004 on aphasia). In this way the person living with dementia together with her or his social network can potentially function as what Hutchins (1995) called a *distributed cognitive system* (Hydén & Forsblad, 2019). As part of this system, the individual living with dementia has access to a much wider number of resources that can be used in the presentation and negotiation of a narrative identity.

This is even true in quite late stages of dementia when the person with dementia has access to very few available resources and is basically unable to tell autobiographical stories on his or her own. If relatives, staff, and others together with the person with dementia are seen as distributed cognitive system, this system can not only provide resources from the life stories but also tell about the person living with dementia. Thus, in the best case, the person with dementia is still part of the storytelling event and his or her autobiographical stories, which define his or her identity, can be told.

Distributed cognitive networks include a re-organization of the interaction between the participants, in order for in particular the person with dementia to make use of the available resources. In the network involving the person with dementia, for instance spouses and family members can take over some of the storytelling functions. This can be accomplished through supporting the person with dementia by helping to identify memories or asking questions at the right point in the telling. When other participants take over interactional and narrative functions, they are also taking over some of the responsibility for the storytelling. This means that the participants without dementia will both have to make more contributions to the storytelling and be more engaged in quite advanced repair work in order for the participant with dementia to continue to be an active conversational participant (Hydén, 2011).

Over time the person living with dementia will slowly lose some of his or her storytelling expertise and hence become more dependent on other persons that can act as "experts" in the storytelling. The person living with dementia may for instance ask the other participant to take over responsibility for the collaboration by asking for help or support. One way of providing support is by creating "scaffolds" that can be used by the person with dementia in order to find words or references or to understand the meaning of contributions made by the other participant (Hydén, 2011). Scaffolds can consist of projected turns formatted in such a way that it will be possible for the person with dementia to use these turns (by using "yes/no" questions for instance). Scaffolds can further consist of often lengthy and complex search activities for words and linguistic expressions as well as for references to past events or persons. The use of these scaffolds will help the person with dementia to continue as an active participant and storyteller by making further contributions to the ongoing storytelling. The narrative scaffolding becomes an integrated part of the ongoing collaboration as a means for joint meaning-making.

Narrative scaffolding is basically directed at keeping an interpersonal relation both by preventing the need for correcting information, as well as "repairing" the storytelling when needed. Narrative scaffolding also aims at protecting the identity of the participant living with dementia and hence their status as a full member of the relation and interaction. By being able to contribute to stories and take part in storytelling it becomes possible for persons with communicative disabilities to continue to be members in interaction.

In conclusion, narrative scaffolding indicates that it is important to include also other persons in the understanding of autobiographic storytelling of persons living with dementia. A focus just on the person with the communicative disability will only capture what the person is able to do without support from other persons. Including also other persons in the analysis and understanding of the person suffering from a stroke will make it clear that storytelling abilities are best described as *socially distributed* abilities, implying that different persons may actually be carrying out various cognitive and linguistic functions. That is, other persons and their abilities can be used as resources for the telling of autobiographical stories and thus maintaining identity.

Using cultural resources: artefacts

As indicated above, cultural resources can be used to construct an identity. One of the most important kinds of cultural resources are storylines, that is, a set of guidelines and constraints for telling a story that conveys it as a story of a certain and recognizable kind (Örulv & Hydén, 2006). Storylines could help a person to sustain a certain narrative about self and thus function as an external support for a personal identity. Other kinds of cultural resources are artefacts that may support identity; photographs might be such a resource.

One context that partly is constructed around the use of storylines is social media. Recently studies have started to explore how people with dementia use social media that also can be utilized as representational structures or resources for narrative identities because the thoughts shared with other people can be understood as the construction of narrative identities. For instance, Talbot et al. (2020; see Thomas, 2017) analysed 2,774 micro texts (tweets) on Twitter from 12 people with dementia and found that themes across participants were most often positive in nature and involved six major narrative themes: nothing about us without us; collective action; experts by experience; living with dementia not suffering from it; community; and stories of dementia. It is significant that the tweets are about a collective illness identity rather than personal experiences. Talbot et al. (2020) argue that tweeting both within and across tweets can be understood as narratives.

Important to understand about any social media is that they scaffold narrative identities. One person was for instance noted to only do so-called retweets (linking other people tweets) and therefore did not produce any tweets by her/himself. However, by retweeting a person can exploit the rich resources of Twitter that have the potential to tap less (or at least other than the faltering) intra-individual cognitive resources; something which becomes necessary when being affected by a dementia disease. The richness of tweets on Twitter together with the retweeting function is a potent resource for creating personal narrative identities based on other people's thoughts and experiences. The parallel to the notion of socially distributed cognition is apparent since it is about someone else carrying out those cognitive and linguistic functions necessary for narrative activity. But what is interesting about social media is that the person with dementia can use other people's functions without knowing them to the extent that is often needed in the co-constructed narrative identities reported on in the previous section where the co-constructor is often a spouse.

Accounts on social media can also function as an external memory of past identity constructions and people with dementia that experience problems with remembering can therefore benefit from being able to return to previous utterances. Something which is not as easily done in analogue real-time constructions of narratives. In such cases the record of past utterances must be co-constructed between the person with dementia and someone who has shared the experience, again most often a spouse.

A study conducted by Karlsson, Zingmark, Axelsson, and Sävenstedt (2017) can be seen a contribution to the understanding of the interaction between the automatically generated records of the past and the analogue real-time constructions of narrative identities. Specifically, they attached a camera to persons with AD that every two minutes automatically generated a photograph of events in front of the person. Photographs were annotated with for instance geolocations and were also grouped in other ways. The photographs with annotation were later used as an elicitation method for narration of recent experiences between the person with AD and a close relative. Indeed, participants were many times helped by the photograph to create co-constructed stories of recent events in relationship to their sense of self. The co-constructions spanned from the person with AD being able to, with little assistance, visualize (project) themselves in(to) the situation the photographs depicted to not being able (without guidance from relatives) to understand the situations depicted. Photographs with people were better prompts than photographs without people and photographs that depicted shared experiences were more easily exploited as a resource in the co-construction of the narratives. The situation was sometimes experienced as being a test situation: knowing that something is a picture of something that one recently experienced can in the presence of others be face-threatening.

In conclusion, when understanding the use of physical objects in narrative identity it is necessary to understand how they anchor thought processes. We can reason that photos of shared experiences can be a powerful co-constructive resource because it is many times something that both contributors of the narrative can perceive as for what it is and demands little imaginative processes. If a physical object is easily perceived for what it is it scaffolds the narrative continuation and allows for the narrative to go beyond the physical and project aspects of an event or process that is not perceivable and hence become a story of the past. The examples above show that this is also possible for people with dementia.

Discussion

Alzheimer's disease and other dementias are fatal, and they change the persons living with the disease. At the same time, it is necessary to learn to live with dementia – and learn to live as well as possible. Emotional pain and memory "loss" is part of dementia, but so is the ability to learn, and the fact that one's self persists and "social memory remains when individual memory falters", as Anne Basting writes (2009, p. 156). This idea of a social memory goes back to the French sociologist Maurice Halbwachs, who argued that "if we examine a little more closely how we recollect things, we will surely realize that the greatest number of memories come back to us when our parents, our friends, or other persons recall them to us" (Halbwachs, 1992, p. 38). In other words, memories and stories are less something "stored" inside the individual mind, and more something that is shared and distributed among people in a person's network. Most autobiographical memories are shared memories that involve other people, and in "remembering" and "recollecting" these memories it is the joint efforts of all these people. When one individual has access to fewer cognitive and linguistic resources due to dementia, the social organization of memories and the joint telling of autobiographical memories become important.

In this chapter we have argued that persons living with dementia as well as their relatives and others, together can attempt to compensate for the diminishing resources available for presenting and negotiating a narrative identity. Regarding the brain resources, people with various forms of dementia can compensate along the semantic–episodic continuum. Important in relationship to this is that it is also the case that normal cognitive ageing involves a change along this continuum. Specifically, there is across the lifespan a trend that people will rely less on their episodic resources and more on their knowledge of the world (Spreng & Turner, 2019). This means that when someone experiences a development of AD typically in old age there are already knowledge of world-resources that would have taken a more central part of narrative identity without the disease.

Further, in several sections above we returned to the various ways co-constructors and the physical environment can scaffold the narrative. In some cases, it is also possible to see that scaffolds work as vehicles of thoughts. For instance, photographs can, when depicting a situation, be tangible in such a way that they tell parts of the story that the person with AD struggles with and therefore make the story more coherent than what it would have been without the photographs. External representations have the power to prove consistency better than humans can do by themselves (Kirsh, 2017) and therefore a photograph and any other cultural resource can act as a source for coherency in narrative identity stories.

Other people can also work as vehicles of thought when telling parts of a story for the person with dementia. What a specific utterance and/or a specific feature of the physical do for narratives for people with dementia are not well-researched. How spouses and others shape the physical environment to structure for people with dementia has been researched in relationship to managing everyday activities (e.g. Hydén, 2014; Majlesi & Ekström, 2016) but has to a lesser extent been researched in relationship to narrative identity. How people close to people with dementia do this naturally and how staff in for instance institutional care do this is not well-researched.

To conclude, it is possible to overcome the challenges that are part of interactional storytelling when having a dementia disease by adopting resources that are available in the brain, in the social surrounding, and the cultural world.

References

Bamberg, M. (2011). Who am I? Narration and its contribution to self and identity. *Theory and Psychology*, 21, 3–24.

Basting, A.D. (2009). *Forget memory: Creating better lives for people with dementia*. Baltimore: Johns Hopkins University Press.

Bitenc, R.A. (2018). "No narrative, no self"? Reconsidering dementia counter-narratives in Tell Mrs Mill Her Husband Is Still Dead. *Subjectivity*, 11, 128–143.

Bratman, M.E. (1992). Shared cooperative activity. *The Philosophical Review*, 101, 327–341.

Brockmeier, J. (2015). *Beyond the archive: Memory, narrative, and the autobiographical process*. New York: Oxford University Press.

Brockmeier, J. & Carbaugh, D. (Eds.) (2001). *Narrative and identity: Studies in autobiography, self and culture*. Amsterdam: John Benjamins.

Bruner, J. (2001). Self-making and world-making. In J. Brockmeier & D. Carbaugh (Eds.), *Narrative and identity: Studies in autobiography, self and culture* (pp. 25–38). Amsterdam: John Benjamins.

Caddell, L.S. & Clare, L. (2010). The impact of dementia on self and identity: A systematic review. *Clinical Psychology Review*, 30, 113–126.

Chafe, W. (1994). *Discourse, consciousness, and time: The flow and displacement of conscious experience in speaking and writing*. Chicago: The University of Chicago Press.

Eustache, M.L., Laisney, M., Juskenaite, A., Letortu, O., Platel, H., Eustache, F., & Desgranges, B. (2013). Sense of identity in advanced Alzheimer's dementia: A cognitive dissociation between sameness and selfhood? *Consciousness and Cognition*, 22, 1456–1467.

Genette, G. (1980). *Narrative discourse: An essay in method*. Ithaca, NY: Cornell University Press.

Gilbert, M. (1990). Walking together: A paradigmatic social phenomenon. *Midwest Studies in Philosophy*, xv, 1–14.

Goodwin, C. (2004). A competent speaker who can't speak: The social life of aphasia. *Journal of Linguistic Anthropology*, 14, 151–170.

Goodwin, C. (2017). *Co-operative action*. New York: Cambridge University Press.

Halbwachs, M. (1992). *On collective memory*. Chicago: University of Chicago Press.

Hollan, J., Hutchins, E., & Kirsh, D. (2000). Distributed cognition: Toward a new foundation for human-computer interaction research. *ACM Transactions on Computer-Human Interaction*, 7, 174–196.

Hutchins, E. (1995). *Cognition in the wild*. Cambridge, MA: MIT Press.

Hydén, L.C. (2008). Broken and vicarious voices in narratives. In L.C. Hydén & J. Brockmeier (Eds.), *Health, culture and illness: Broken narratives* (pp. 36–53). New York: Routledge.

Hydén, L.C. (2011). Narrative collaboration and scaffolding in dementia. *Journal of Aging Studies*, 25, 339–347.

Hydén, L.C. (2014). Cutting Brussels sprouts: Collaboration involving persons with dementia. *Journal of Aging Studies*, 29, 115–123.

Hydén, L.C. (2018). *Entangled narratives: Collaborative storytelling and the re-imagining of dementia*. New York: Oxford University Press.

Hydén, L.C. (2020). Dementia and identity. In M. Bamberg, C. Demuth, & M. Watzlawik (Eds.), *Cambridge handbook of identity*. New York: Cambridge University.

Hydén, L.C. & Brockmeier, J. (Eds.) (2008). *Health, culture and illness: Broken narratives*. New York: Routledge.

Hydén, L.C. & Forsblad, M. (2019). Collaborative remembering in dementia: The perspective from activity theory. In M. Meade, C.B. Harris, P. Van Bergen, J. Sutton, & A.J. Barnier (Eds.), *Collaborative remembering: Theories, research, and applications*. Oxford: Oxford University Press.

Karlsson, E., Zingmark, K., Axelsson, K., & Sävenstedt, S. (2017). Aspects of self and identity in narrations about recent events: Communication with individuals with Alzheimer's disease enabled by a digital photograph diary. *Journal of Gerontological Nursing*, 43(6), 25–31.

Kirsh, D. (2017). Thinking with external representations. In S.J. Cowley & F. Vallée-Tourangeau (Eds.), *Cognition beyond the brain: Computation, interactivity and human artifice* (pp. 171–194). London: Springer.

Labov, W. (1972). The transformation of experience in narrative syntax. In W. Labov, *Language in the inner city* (pp. 354–405). Philadelphia: University of Pennsylvania Press.

Lezak, M.D., Howieson, D.B., Bigler, E.D., & Tranel, D. (2012). *Neuropsychological assessment* (5th Edition). New York: Oxford University Press.

Luria, A.R. (1973). *The working brain: An introduction to neuropsychology*. Harmondsworth: Allen Lane The Penguin Press.

McAdams, D.P. (2006). *The redemptive self: Stories Americans live by*. New York: Oxford University Press.

McAdams, D.P., Josselson, R., & Lieblich, A. (Eds.) (2001). *Turns in the road: Narrative studies of lives in transition*. Seattle: APA.

McKeown, J., Clarke, A., & Repper, J. (2006). Life story work in health and social care: Systematic literature review. *Journal of Advanced Nursing*, 55, 237–247.

Majlesi, A.R. & Ekström, A. (2016). Baking together: The coordination of actions in activities involving people with dementia. *Journal of Aging Studies*, 38, 37–46.

Mar, R.A. (2004). The neuropsychology of narrative: Story comprehension, story production and their interrelation. *Neuropsychologia*, 42, 1414–1434.

Ochs, E. & Capps, L. (2001). *Living narrative: Creating lives in everyday storytelling*. Cambridge, MA: Harvard University Press.

Örulv, L. & Hydén, L.C. (2006). Confabulation: Sense-making, self-making and world-making in dementia. *Discourse Studies*, 8, 647–673.

Perkins, M. (2007). *Pragmatic impairment*. Cambridge: Cambridge University Press.

Shenk, D., Davis, B., Peacock, J.R., & Moore, L. (2002). Narratives and self-identity in later life: Two rural American older women. *Journal of Aging Studies*, 16, 401–413.

Spreng, R.N. & Turner, G.R. (2019). The shifting architecture of cognition and brain function in older adulthood. *Perspectives on Psychological Science*, 14, 523–542.

Strikwerda-Brown, C., Grilli, M.D., Andrews-Hanna, J., & Irish, M. (2019). "All is not lost": Rethinking the nature of memory and the self in dementia. *Ageing Research Reviews*, 54. doi:10.1016/j.arr.2019.100932.

Surr, C.A. (2006). Preservation of self in people with dementia living in residential care: A socio-biographical approach. *Social Science and Medicine*, 62, 1720–1730.

Talbot, C.V., O'Dwyer, S.T., Clare, L., Janet, H., & Anderson, J. (2020). How people with dementia use Twitter: A qualitative analysis. *Computers in Human Behavior*, 102, 112–119.

Thomas, B. (2017). Whose story is it anyway: Following everyday accounts of living with dementia on social media. *Style*, 51, 357–373.

Wilson, S.M., Henry, M.L., Besbris, M., Ogar, J.M., Dronkers, N.F., Jarrold, W., & Gorno-Tempini, M.L. (2010). Connected speech production in three variants of primary progressive aphasia. *Brain*, 133, 2069–2088.

6 Recovery stories of people diagnosed with severe mental illness

Katabatic and anabatic narratives

Francisco Javier Saavedra-Macías

Illness narratives (INs) are considered a genre with idiosyncratic features that have had an impact even on the history of literature. In this chapter, we defend the existence of another parallel genre of narratives in the field of mental health: those we could call *recovery narratives* (RNs). In the first section, we will describe narratives as essential tools through which we construct our identity. We will define INs and describe their functions. In the second section, we will offer some of the classifications of INs and briefly explore their characteristics in the specific field of mental illness, in literature and in contemporary culture. In the third section, we will explain the model of recovery in mental health and its scientific, professional, and political repercussions. Finally, in the fourth section, we define and describe the characteristics of RNs and provide examples.

Identity, narrative, and illness

From a biomedical perspective, illness is described as a biological imbalance. Thus, our body is objectified and demystified to the extent that it is stripped of any meaning that distinguishes it from other bodies, deprived of any sign of personification. In this sense, the metaphor of the broken machine is a very appropriate simile.

However, illness, especially when it is chronic or severe – for example, a diagnosis of schizophrenia – represents a break in the patient's biography, a break in his or her identity. Illness transforms our body; it causes us pain; it alters the body's functions and makes our daily activities difficult or impossible; it alters the perception of basic categories such as time and space; it changes our personal relationships and inevitably forces us to question who we are. A serious illness represents a break between our body, the world around us, and our self. In short, a serious illness demands that we rework our identity (Bury, 1982).

The classic differentiation between *disease, illness*, and *sickness* made by Kleinman (1988) is an attempt to distinguish and highlight this subjective dimension of illness from the biological framework. To Kleinman, the term *disease* refers to the biological dimension of the illness. Thus, the concept of *disease* is what the professional sees through the lens of the scientific discipline in which he or she has been trained. On the contrary, the term *illness* includes the perceptions, explanations, evaluations, emotions, types of coping, expectations, judgements, etc., not only of the sick person, but also of their families and loved ones. Therefore, cultural factors must always be considered when we want to understand the experience of illness, since its meaning – beyond its biological aetiology – is the core. Finally, Kleinman uses the term *sickness* to refer to illness when considering political, economic, or institutional factors in large populations.

We organize our experiences through the narratives that we tell about ourselves, giving them cultural meanings and making them communicable. The narrative is the basic tool that allows us to construct our identities. In this sense, a narrative is the canonical form in which we communicate our experiences of illness; so much so that, in society, a coherent and shareable narrative about oneself is a necessary condition for social recognition (Saavedra, 2009b). Therefore, narratives should be understood as an empirical phenomenon articulated in communicative actions of a subject faced with the task of giving an account of his or her life in specific situations (Lucius-Hoene & Deppermann, 2002). One of these extraordinary situations will undoubtedly be the diagnosis of an illness. We will now comment very briefly on the properties of life narratives (self-narratives).

According to some psychologists (Bruner, 1991), they can be understood as cognitive instruments of a semiotic and therefore cultural nature. Two planes coexist in all narratives: the plane of action where facts and actions are described, and the plane of consciousness where our subjective experiences develop. Through narratives, we express or discover projects, the consequences of an action, emotions, hidden thoughts (sometimes contradictory to an action). Therefore, narratives are essential in order to communicate human drama, to be able to get inside the minds of others (theory of mind) and to understand their doubts and contradictions. Due to the sequential nature of language and, therefore, narratives, it is possible to organize the events of our life and the experience of time. Besides being cognitive tools, narratives are linguistic actions that are always constructed within the framework of social interactions. The social nature of narratives can be observed clearly when we find established discursive models or genres in them. These help us to construct our stories in a more acceptable way within specific communities.

As we have seen above, narratives are actions, but they also contain descriptions of actions. Thus, they can explore the narrator's capacity for agency on two planes. On the one hand, within the narrative, seeing whether the narrator describes him or herself as a person with the capacity to influence the world around them, with the capacity to control events; or if the narrator simply shows him or herself as a passive being, facing various forces outside of their control. On the other hand, if the narrator, by means of the very action of the narration, is transforming their own life story thanks to the strategic use of the semiotic tools that we have mentioned above (structure of events, causal relations, emotions employed, use of discursive genres, etc.). Therefore, the use of narratives can be considered a way to take control of our experiences. In one of the most fruitful and astonishing autobiographical works on illness, Anatole Broyard explains why he decided to write about his experiences as a coping strategy:

> I'm not a doctor, and even as a patient I'm a mere beginner. Yet I am a critic, and being critically ill, I thought I might accept the pun and turn it on my condition. My initial experience of illness was a series of disconnected shocks, and my first instinct was to try to get it under control by turning it into a narrative. In emergency situations we always invent narratives. We describe what is happening, as if this would allow us to confine the catastrophe ... Storytelling seems to be a natural reaction to the illness. People bleed stories, and I've become a blood bank of them.
>
> (Broyard, 2013, p. 42)

Narratives, especially autobiographical ones, always have a moral component by which the audience becomes an authority that grants acceptance or rejection. The final goal of a narrative is very concrete: to give an account of the current situation of a subject in the world (Saavedra, 2009b). In other words, it seeks to justify or make understandable some specific experiences in a community, to make them communicable. In this case, a narrative whose main theme is a serious illness, such as a diagnosis of a serious mental disorder, and whose author is a patient – although family members or professionals should also be considered – would try to answer the following questions: How did I come to suffer from these problems? How was it possible for me to be diagnosed with this illness? Therefore, narratives – and, among these, INs – always have an ethical or moral plane (Ricoeur, 1987).

Hydén (1997) summarizes the characteristics of INs that we have noted above into five functions or uses:

1 The narratives give new signs and a new structure for rebuilding a world that has been broken down by illness. Thus, experiences can be articulated and shared again.
2 Thanks to these new signs and the new articulation of experiences, narratives allow us to revise our personal identities and our life stories in terms of illness and to negotiate new reasons.
3 Narratives allow us to explore possible explanations for the illness. Possible explanations or causes for the illness may be related to our moral values and our lifestyles. Thus, according to Hydén, narratives become a "moral tester". The different aetiologies we use to explain our experiences can also determine the coping modes we use to fight the illness.
4 According to the pragmatic nature of language, narratives can be used as strategic tools to achieve different objectives. For example, they can be used to justify actions, to gain some recognition, to ask for help, to gain authority, etc.
5 Finally, through narratives we transform our private experiences into collective experiences. In this way, we can take part in political and social contexts. In this sense, narratives of patients with severe mental illness (SMIs) have been fundamental in building a political and social community that defends their rights as citizens.

Illness narratives: madness in literature and culture

There are various categorizations of INs in the field of psychological disorders. For example, Lysaker and Lysaker (2002) propose three types of categories based on the analysis of the dialogical relationships between different positions within the narratives of people diagnosed with schizophrenia: cacophonous, monological, and empty. The adjective *cacophonous* denotes a fracture of dialogue since the person is filled with an amalgam of I-positions, with no hierarchy or organization. In this way, people are incapable of constructing an identity with socially accepted meaning. *Monological* refers to a single I-position that dominates the narration. This control makes it impossible to change the narrative and can eventually lead to psychotic symptoms like delusions. The term *empty* concerns a lack of the dialogical capacity between I-positions and others from the social world. Saavedra, Cubero, and Crawford (2009) added a fourth type of narrative in people with schizophrenia: *complexity and articulation of narratives*. These narratives show a complex narrative pattern with connections amongst I-positions and others from the social world.

Frank (1995) and Robinson (1990) created other classifications based on narrative structure. The former divided INs into three categories: "restitution", "chaos", and "quest". The second, in a similar vein, suggested three types of INs: stable, progressive, and regressive.

Hydén (1997), by analysing the relationship between the narrator, the narrative, and the illness, proposes the following taxonomy: illness as narrative, narrative about illness, and narrative as illness. Due to the originality of this proposal, we will briefly define each of these categories. In the first case, the narrator, the illness, and the narrative are merged in the same person. Thus, the narrative is the way in which the narrator articulates and expresses the experiences of illness. This type of INs would correspond to the proposal described in the extract from Broyard (2013) presented earlier. The integration of symptoms, expectations, emotions, explanations, etc., structured in the same narrative would create a new *social reality*, a new *world of illness*, according to Hydén (1997). In other words, INs not only represent reality: they construct it. In the case of *narratives about illness*, they become a transmission belt for clinical knowledge and ideas about illness. An example could be those stories about patients written by professionals. Therefore, narratives become an essential training tool for health professionals and, of course, a tool to build medical science itself. Various authors such as Sacks (1985) and Charon (2001) maintain that health professionals should be experts in their patients' narratives, not only as a means of delving deeper into their pathological features, but also to be able to communicate effectively with the patients and optimize personal encounters and treatment. Finally, *narratives as illness* become a sign of the illness themselves. For example, the narratives of a patient suffering from paranoid delusions, or the stories of a person with dementia who makes up part of his life. In these cases, the narratives do not have the complexity, coherence, and minimal structure that makes them interpretable and able to be shared in the community. The *cacophonous* and *monological* categories proposed by Lysaker and Lysaker

(2002) can be included in Hydén's classification. Clearly, narratives as illness would not have the five functions we mentioned at the end of the previous section.

Something that we believe is important to add to Hydén's taxonomy (1997), and which is perhaps not sufficiently emphasized, is that these types of narratives are not incompatible. That is to say, it may be the case that a narrative belongs at the same time to the categories *narratives as illness* and *narratives about illness.* For example, a patient with a clinical background may write about his or her illness, so the perspectives of the professional and the patient would intersect in the story. In Carol North's memoirs (1990), *Welcome, Silence: My Triumph over Schizophrenia*, the author narrates her experiences with illness from secondary school to hospital admissions, interspersed with her perspective as a psychiatrist. On the other hand, patients with psychological disorders who construct narratives about their illness are sometimes still symptomatically active and their delusions or hallucinations invade their stories. Nevertheless, the symptoms do not always annul the social meaning of these stories, although they may make them difficult to interpret (Saavedra et al., 2009).

Falconer (2005) points to a common set of characteristics in the memoirs of people who have suffered mental illness, i.e. their INs. One of these characteristics is the use of metaphors referencing the works of Dante and Lewis Carroll – and in some cases, direct references to them. Allusions to these authors and the use of images such as hell, the descent into the underworld, or crossing the mirror relate the experience of illness to a breakdown of the established symbolic world, and at times, to the moral and socio-economic framework of Western societies. A clear example of the use of these metaphors in the narratives of people diagnosed with schizophrenia and other psychoses is found in *Asylum Piece* by Anna Kavan (1940). This author relies on her traumatic admissions to psychiatric hospitals to describe in third person the emptiness and objectification of institutionalized life. This breakdown of the symbolic world has been considered the essential characteristic of how the experience of the self is altered in schizophrenia (Lysaker et al., 2018). As Falconer (2005) also states, the experience of mental illness reflects the most intimate nightmare of Western industrialized societies: the threat to the ultimate societal achievement, the breakdown of a stable, essential, and autonomous self. This self had been built up from the Renaissance, and later the Enlightenment and the Industrial Revolution, to the present day. In fact, we can find descriptions of hallucinatory experiences that include images of the collapse of the contemporary industrial world in some testimonies of people with SMIs. For example, Haire (2008) describes her experience with illness in an autobiographical account of her abuse, rape, and journey into psychosis. In the following excerpt, in which she tells us about her psychotic symptoms, Haire combines images of hell with descriptions of catastrophes that come from the industrial-capitalist imaginary:

> I know flames and fires featured a lot in my hallucinations and I have since wondered if all this was a symbolic representation of all the anger I had suppressed in my life. The energy rush of the psychosis was quite

> incredible – almost orgasmic, but in a sinister sort of way. Some of the imagery will stay in my mind forever, of distorted bodies trapped in a huge net at the bottom of the sea, or the collapse of an oil rig; of Siamese twins and severed limbs. There was also the feeling of travelling at speed on a fast rollercoaster, of being hurled from this rollercoaster at a fairground, of imagining I was pregnant too. Bubbling oil and oil rigs often featured in the hallucinations and the oil rig was on the verge of collapse.
>
> (Haire, 2008, p. 87)

Not surprisingly, in line with the theological and mythological images, ideas of identity possession and fragmentation are frequent in these narratives. For example, in his autobiographical account of his experiences with his teenage daughter, who was diagnosed with bipolar disorder, Greenberg (2008) honestly and movingly explores this metaphor, possession, as a possible explanation for his daughter's transformation:

> With each question I await a response, the slightest indication that whatever spell she is under has broken and she is the child I know again. Each time, however, her otherness is reaffirmed. It is as if the real Sally has been kidnapped, and here in her place is a demon, like Solomon's, who has appropriated her body. The ancient superstition of possession! How else to come to grips with this grotesque transformation?
>
> (Greenberg, 2008, p. 29)

The figure of the double or Doppelgänger, according to the expression coined by Jean Paul, is a long-standing tradition in literature and reflects the features of many narratives of people suffering from SMIs (Saavedra & Vélez, 2011). The heroes of this literary genre, cultivated by authors as dissimilar as Hoffman, Dostoyevsky, or Saramago, fear that they will be swallowed up by the outside world and that others may get inside their minds. These characters yearn for contact with the social world but are terrified of the idea that this physical and emotional contact will fragment them and end up destroying their fragile identity. They feel as if they live in a post-modern Dante's inferno, that they are automatons or that they have the power to transform others into automatons. The identity of the heroes in these novels is always threatened by fragmentation, as are the identities and narratives of the people diagnosed with SMI who have told us about their lives (Saavedra & Vélez, 2011; Lysaker & Lysaker, 2002).

Falconer (2005) describes three representations of "hell" in the published autobiographical narratives of people with severe mental illness. On the one hand, the different health care institutions are analogous to hell in these narratives. Thus, involuntary hospitalization in psychiatric hospitals and daily life in them have been described as a descent into hell. Falconer offers the example of Linda Hart's *Phone at Nine Just to Say You are Alive* (1997), in which she describes the hospital where she was admitted as a hell with several kingdoms, upper and lower, like Dante's hell. A second representation of hell in patients' narratives are the specific symptoms they experience. Marya Hornbacher (1998), in her autobiographical work *Wasted: A Memoir of Anorexia and Bulimia*, describes her bulimia symptoms – of which she is both victim and perpetrator – as hell.

Finally, Falconer identifies a third model in which hell is represented in the INs of people with SMIs. In this model, hell becomes a copy of the path taken by the narrator in the descent into the depths of his or her traumas, the source of the narrator's psychosis. Falconer notes that frequently the authors of INs have a friend, doctor, or family member who accompanies them on their journey, just as Dante had Virgil as a guide on his descent into the underworld. Hart's narrative, *Phone at Nine Just to Say You are Alive*, may serve as an example. In this case, the journey is a trip back in memory to find the core of the trauma. As a guide on her journey to the underworld, Linda Hart has the help of a friend who had survived a psychological disorder as well. This friend could be called a "peer supporter". It is worth noting that peer support programmes are a pillar of the new organization of health and social services in the framework of recovery. That is to say, including in the services the help of people diagnosed with SMIs who are in the process of recovery as guides and support for people with first episodes of illness.

Falconer (2005) treats these narratives as a specific literary genre by framing them in what she calls the *katabatic tradition*. The term "katabasis" refers to the descent to the underworld by heroes in Ancient Greece. With this descent into the underworld as the core of these narratives, Falconer states that, in all of them, the return from hell depends on an "inversion of perspective", "a clarification and reorientation of values", necessarily entailing "an affirmation of the everyday, material world". At this point, in the following section, we would like to introduce and develop the premises of the recovery model in mental health in order to, in the fourth and last section, propose the existence of another genre in the field of mental health, which parallels the one described by Falconer and was born fostered by the recovery movement: "*recovery narratives*" (RNs).

Recovery model in mental health

Since the second half of the twentieth century, it has been acknowledged that adequate treatment of mental health problems must address not only the symptomatological aspects, but also the behavioural and social ones. In short, understanding mental illness requires a broad perspective from integrative models. The concepts of rehabilitation and integration guided mental health care programmes in the last century, with the aim of providing patients with SMIs with the resources and skills needed to become integrated citizens in society. In the 1990s, a new model of mental health care burst onto the scene. Although it was slightly related to previous models, this new form revolutionized intervention practices and programmes, and was called the recovery model (Saavedra, 2011). Today, it is the prevailing model, at least on paper, in the mental health systems of Anglo-Saxon countries. It is also very influential in the countries of Southern Europe, although its explicit presence has less of an impact. The recovery model originates in narratives and autobiographies, and in the subjective experiences of the affected people – these describe their recovery processes. These stories show us that it is possible to achieve a meaningful and socially connected life. Therefore, movements led by the affected people and social rights initiatives are the reason why the concept of recovery has been brought closer to our mental health system (Jacobson & Curtis, 2000). The position of these groups is, in some cases, very belligerent with the psychiatric care system, to the extent that they refer to themselves as survivors of the system.

According to a classic definition (Anthony, 1993), recovery is a process specific to each person, and it requires reconstructing the identity with the aim of developing, despite the illness, new meanings and purposes to achieve a meaningful life. Another more contemporary and comprehensive definition of the recovery model is offered by the Sainsbury Centre for Mental Health. This institution describes recovery as a set of values about a person's rights to build a meaningful life for themselves, with or without the continued presence of mental health symptoms. Recovery is based on the ideas of self-determination and self-control. It emphasizes the importance of hope in maintaining motivation, as well as receiving help to achieve a meaningful life (The Future Vision Coalition, 2009, p. 22).

The definition of what recovery means may vary depending on where we put our focus and the context from which we make the definition (e.g. professionals or people affected). However, according to Lerany, Bird, Williams, and Slade (2011) in a review of over 5,000 papers on recovery, there are five common psychosocial processes in all recovery processes: connectedness, hope and optimism about the future, identity, meaning in life, and empowerment.

The recovery model has led to the reform of mental health services in a way that is almost opposite to services oriented to the treatment or cure from a strictly bio-health perspective. Recovery-oriented services promote the empowerment and control of users in their interactions with health and social services (The Future Vision Coalition, 2009). Since the beginning of the twenty-first century, it is easy to find guidelines for the implementation of recovery-oriented services in Ireland, England, the United States, and other Western countries. Among other proposals, we can see the inclusion of users or affected people in professional teams, the creation of care contracts in which affected people negotiate the treatment with professionals and new interdisciplinary teams. We can also find a growing participation of users and affected people in the political commissions that make decisions regarding the management of the mental health system.

The model of recovery in mental health entails several challenges for the classic health systems. To begin with, many of the key objectives of recovery are qualitative and subjective in nature and depend entirely on the individual's perspective. Therefore, the measurement, evaluation, and study of recovery is problematic because it is very difficult or impossible to make it a target. For this reason, the model of recovery has promoted qualitative research on the narratives of affected people. Also, the recovery model is committed to designing programmes in which affected people increasingly take control of their treatment and care plans, including intervening at the organizational and political levels. Obviously, this fact forces us to rethink professional practices in the field of mental health, for example, "peer support" programmes that involve the inclusion of affected people in work teams in mental health institutions. Finally, this model assumes that recovery is possible without treatment and that some people can freely choose not to use mental health services. In other words, it states that recovery from a psychological disorder is not necessarily related to the services, programmes, and professionals that are theoretically intended for it (Slade & Longden, 2015).

RNs have become so relevant that it is possible to find official guides for their creation and distribution. Some of the institutions that publish guides for constructing RNs are the Scottish Recovery Network, the Mental Health Commission of Canada, and associations such as Mind in the UK (Llewellyn-Beardsley et al., 2019; Woods, Hart, & Spandler, 2019). Among these institutions, we can highlight the "Recovery Colleges". These are educational centres created specifically with the purpose of promoting recovery, and one of their activities is providing training for the creation and dissemination of RNs. The first Recovery College was founded in South West London in 2009, and the second shortly after, in Nottingham. Today, there are several dozen Recovery Colleges operating in England, Scotland, Australia, and other countries.

In the following section, we will describe in detail the characteristics of RNs. We will argue that they can be considered as a specific, related, but independent genre of the INs we have discussed previously.

Recovery narratives

Interest in RNs is growing. Several systematic reviews on RNs have recently been published (Rennick-Egglestone et al., 2019; Llewellyn-Beardsley et al., 2019; Slade et al., 2012). Next, we will highlight (although not exhaustively) the narrative characteristics of the recovery stories that we consider essential and that we find both in scientific literature and in online institutional resources.

Individual authorship

An essential feature of RNs is their individual authorship. In other words, recovery is the product of a personal process carried out in the first person. Therefore, narratives are individual creations of the people affected. Family members and professionals can be authors in the genre of INs, as we have seen above, but first-person authorship is a priority. However, RNs are exclusively produced by affected people.

Although the associative movement was key in the emergence of the recovery model – as we have previously indicated – collective narratives are secondary. In fact, recovery is essentially described as an inner transformation, a change of perspective and patterns, a process of empowerment leading to personal fulfilment. Llewellyn-Beardsley et al. (2019) call this narrative format "enlightenment". Woods, Hart, and Spandler (2019) argue that RNs can be called an "insight or inspiring genre" insofar as, in order to be effective, they generate a transformation of the self; they must be shared, publicly exposed, thus turning the audience (possible interlocutors or readers) into witnesses and, paradoxically, final arbiters of the recovery. Llewellyn-Beardsley et al. (2019) describe the existence of "turning points", in the sense developed by Bruner (1991), in RNs. In these episodes, which are sometimes traumatic in nature, a renewed awareness of the experience is achieved. These moments can be called epiphanic, in the sense that they reveal a new reality and lead to post-traumatic growth (Slade & Longden, 2015). On this matter, illness, in an extreme way, can be understood as a gift that transforms the subject's identity. In the following excerpt, a 46-year-old woman diagnosed with bipolar disorder explains how she would refer to her psychological problems in a job interview:

> What I would say is that … well, that I have many resources, that I am a very hard working person, and that for the position I have applied to, my mental disability, no, it is not a problem, it is more, I think, of a gift. I am convinced that it is a gift, and that I can make the illness go away, so I think it is a luxury to have an illness.

Without a doubt, social connection is a dimension of recovery that exists in all definitions of recovery. However, it is not a defining feature of these narratives, and on many occasions the social dimension is described more as a sphere of influence of recovery than as an explanatory key to it. For example, in the exhaustive analysis by Llewellyn-Beardsley et al. (2019) of 629 "recovery narratives" belonging to 49 studies, only two of these took into account the sociocultural dimension. For these reasons, some scholars have coined the term "relational model of recovery" as opposed to the "self model of recovery" in order to emphasize the interpersonal nature of recovery processes (Price-Robertson, Obradovic, & Morgan, 2016; Price-Robertson, Manderson, & Duff, 2017).

Agency

Another fundamental feature of these narratives is the capacity of agency of the protagonist of the story. The narrators of these stories, after the turning point we mentioned earlier, make decisions, carry out actions, and intervene in their environment (McAdams & Bowman, 2001). In short, they become agents who face problems and conflicts instead of being passive subjects of the actions of health and family. In narrative terms, the active voice is frequently used, and the appearance of action verbs, such as "I decided", "I did", "I studied", "I learned", is common. Logically, obstacles do not disappear from the narratives, but the narrator focuses on the much or little agency that he or she has, leaving in the background the context and the circumstances that limit the narrator. For example, medication can be described as a disease management resource that is negotiated with health professionals. On the contrary, from a position without agency, taking medication could be described as a medical order, considered a sign of illness, something that the narrator takes passively and causes numerous setbacks.

Thus, in addition to being essentially individual in nature, RNs are described by their authors as agents and autonomous. In the following excerpt, which is taken from the narrative of a 32-year-old unemployed man with a severe mental disorder, the agency and autonomy typical of the recovery genre can be observed. In the text, the interviewee explains what it means for him to have lost his job:

> You have time to reflect and try and change things … you're laid off and you say to yourself: "Right. Why have I been laid off?" So you think about it and come to a conclusion. And so this can stir up your ambitions, it can wake you up, make you want to move, because I want more than I've got here. I'm going to this company even though it will be harder because that is the objective I'm going to set myself. You set yourself an objective.
>
> (Saavedra, López, González, & Cubero, 2016)

Upward trajectory

In contrast to INs, Llewellyn-Beardsley et al. (2019) conducted a systematic review of studies, in which they found that the most frequently described structure in RNs is a bottom-up approach. These narratives can be described as "narratives of revelation or purposeful suffering". We could use the term "anabatic" in this framework, which means ascending or growing. The redemptive self, described by McAdams (2008), fits perfectly into this type of ascending narrative in the genre of recovery. The redemptive self is, according to McAdams, a prototype of a hero who faces obstacles and suffering until he manages to "transform evil into good" with moral certainty and courage. The construction of this self as an agent in narratives of upward trajectories has a great persuasive power in the framework of the North American culture in particular, and Anglo-Saxon culture in general (McAdams, 2008). However, these same authors (Llewellyn-Beardsley et al., 2019) and others (Saavedra, 2009a) describe narratives in which there are no dramatic experiences of healing and recovery – there are stories of endurance, marked by failures and small moments of happiness based on everyday experiences.

Goal-directed

As we have seen, narratives have the purpose of organizing the episodes of our lives in order to account for life itself. INs try to give meaning to episodes of illness. But RNs, contrary to INs, must project into the future. RNs cannot simply provide a coherent and cohesive account of the past; they must also set objectives and imagine the future. From a cognitive perspective, some authors have called future episodic memory or future episodic thinking the capacity to imagine our future, and they have argued that the same system of episodic memory allows us to represent the past and the future (Schacter & Addis, 2007). In the following excerpt, we can see how a 50-year-old man diagnosed with schizophrenia describes his future in his life narrative:

> I imagine my future as getting up early, going to work, going out at two or three in the afternoon and then in the afternoon being around the house, helping out, and also having a little time, even if it's two hours, well, to write and read, for my projects … Andalusian culture really appeals to me, and I have the project of writing, well I already had my degree project on that, so I want to make it bigger and publish it.

Emotional nature

As we saw at the beginning of the chapter, narratives always present a subjective plane, the plane of consciousness, which has a contextual and always situated value. As opposed to narrative thinking, in paradigmatic thinking we find propositions that relate to each other based on universal logical-mathematical laws (Bruner, 1991). At the subjective or conscious plane, we can frame emotions, which are essential to any narrative construction.

Despite the significance of this subjective plane in all narratives, we can also find logical arguments, appeals to authority, formulation of hypotheses, presentation of laws, or description of facts. However, in the genre of recovery, due to its individual and subjective nature, every element of paradigmatic thinking, according to Bruner's definition (1991), is overlooked by the most subjective aspects, such as emotions. Appeals to scientific evidence, the use of psychological or psychiatric terminology, appeals to professional authority, the use of scientific models to explain experiences, etc., are secondary to the personal and emotional experience of the author of the narrative, where all his or her authority and rhetorical force lie. In this sense, the description of pain, uncertainty, and distress due to illness, professional treatment or social norms, resistance, and struggle in pursuit of recovery, and subsequent rebirth or advancement are key to understanding the genre of recovery. Recently, the expression of emotional experiences in RNs has been identified as a potential stress factor for recipients (Rennick-Egglestone et al., 2019).

Some authors have provocatively used the term "recovery porn" to critically discuss inflation and the pressure to build RNs where intimate experiences (emotions) with mental illness are publicly exposed and then used uncontrollably by institutions and individuals outside the survivors' movement (Costa et al., 2012).

Moral and political function

Every narrative has a moral function, even a political one, since they try to explain and justify our position in the world, our identity. Taking this statement as true, there are narratives whose moral burden is more intense, since they are directly related to how we should construct our identity. RNs have been categorized as a "technology of recovery" (Woods et al., 2019) in the sense that the very fact of constructing and sharing them facilitates recovery. Therefore, they can also be called a "genre of insight", since through them we build a way of behaving and understanding our experiences and the world. Furthermore, the functions of these narratives when promoted by various institutions – from public administration, associations, or health institutions – are almost endless. According to these authors, RNs are tools in anti-stigma campaigns, in fundraising, in psychosocial and clinical education, in health policy reform, in promoting new therapeutic practices or in achieving the objectives of groups of survivors, etc.

Woods et al. (2019) warn us against assuming that expressing experiences with mental illness through this genre is "inherently" positive. Along these lines, some authors have pointed out the various kinds of harm that may result from sharing experiences with mental illness within the framework of the recovery genre in an uncritical way (Costa et al., 2012; Voronka, 2016).

Conclusions

According to Bakhtin (1987), a stereotyped use of a series of linguistic statements with a common style and objectives in a given historical moment shows the existence of a discursive genre. Similarly, Gergen and Gergen (1986) assert that there are narrative forms widely shared in society with specific purposes. In this sense, we maintain that there is a narrative genre of recovery that is intimately related to mental health, but whose presence can be explored in other areas of health. Moreover, the persuasive power and presence in different institutions and media of these narratives allows them to be called "master narratives". According to McAdams and McLean (2013), the master narratives are a product of social practices and privileged discourses in interactive scenarios. These narratives are characteristics of a particular cultural group. They are sociocultural artefacts and are essential for socialization. The "master narratives" intervene in basic psychological processes, such as memory, operating as basic schemes that guide the recovery of information (Arias-Sánchez, Saavedra, Santamaría, & Smorti, 2019).

We may wonder whether RNs belong to a totally different genre than the INs we described at the beginning of this chapter, or whether they can be considered a sub-genre of the latter. In trying to apply Hydén's taxonomy of INs (1997) to RNs, we find that it is not a perfect fit. On the one hand, "recovery as narratives" and "narratives as recovery" would merge, since the very act of building a RN and sharing it would somehow involve a positive transformation of its author.

On the other hand, "narratives about recovery" would be put in a paradoxical situation. The latter require the distancing and systematization of the recovery experience – often from a professional or scientific perspective – which would detract from the authority of these narratives and contradict the unique and non-transferable nature of the recovery process.

There are numerous features which separate, as defined by Kleinman (1988) and Frank (1995), from those of recovery. For example, we can find recovery outside the health system in RNs, thus challenging the power of psychiatric diagnosis as a framework of meaning (Llewellyn-Beardsley et al., 2019). The most differentiating feature between both narrative genres is probably the existence of the anabasis stage or upward trajectory, which is central in RNs and optional in INs. The use of metaphors such as "gift" to refer to the illness, in contrast to the metaphors of descent common to INs (which we describe in the second section) is a characteristic of this upward trajectory. RNs are, without any doubt, a field of study that is in its infancy when compared to INs, which have a century of theoretical study.

The proliferation of RNs has led to a critical review of them and a preliminary assessment of their impact on recipients. Even possible negative impacts of RNs on their recipients have been tentatively described (Rennick-Egglestone et al., 2019). Some of the grey areas of RNs that have been described are the individual bias that marginalizes the political, social, and cultural sphere as an explanatory factor (Price-Robertson et al., 2016); their marked Anglo-Saxon cultural nature and the absence of studies in other cultures (Slade et al., 2012); the growing homogeneity of these narratives, which makes it difficult for other narrative structures and content to be visible; the pressure from institutions, media, and social groups to build these types of narratives; and the political and institutional use of these narratives without the due control of their authors (Costa et al., 2012; Voronka, 2016; Woods et al., 2019).

As Broyard (2013) states, each person should construct his or her own style of facing the illness and, we add, a style to create his or her own path to recovery:

> The genre of illness should have a literary critic … who would speak in defence of the therapeutic values of the style, since it seems to me that any seriously ill person should develop a style that is specific to the illness. I believe that only if one insists on their style will they be able to save themselves from falling out of love with themselves when the illness tries to diminish or disfigure them. Sometimes vanity is the only thing that keeps us alive, and one's style is the instrument that vanity uses.
>
> (Broyard, 2013, p. 49)

RNs are an essential instrument for constructing new meanings to live a full life, in spite of or against illness. There is ample scientific evidence of the influence of meaning and coherence not only on the quality of life and psychological well-being, but also on the physiological response to stress. However, the overwhelming success and institutionalization of a narrative genre that is too restricted could make other narratives invisible, and even put the blame on people who do not have the resources to reproduce that genre or, as stated by Broyard, to have a style of their own. From our perspective, the danger lies in the influence of some type of transcendentalism, individualistic and idealistic by definition, in the model of recovery. Recovery perceived as a moral imperative, the product of a mainly subjective effort, is what could shift the model away from the recovery of scientific and social premises and bring it closer to pseudo-sciences. Some authors have described the uncritical production and inclusion of "happy ends" and false expectations in the narratives we consume due to social and institutional pressures as "cruel optimism" (Berlant, 2011) or "näive hope" (McAdams, 2008). Regarding narratives of the "redemptive self", McAdams states:

> There is no perfect life narrative, just as there is no perfect life, or perfect society. Every narrative identity is like a double-edged sword, cutting both ways. The redemptive self affirms a generative commitment to society, but it opens itself up to the dangers of psychological and cultural exceptionalism. The redemptive self celebrates the power of human resilience and growth, but it may also fall prey to arrogance and self-righteousness. The redemptive self sustains hope, but blind hope is naïve.
>
> (McAdams, 2008, p. 26)

We must remember that, although narratives are instruments of identity construction and new meanings, they do not change reality by themselves. There is no narrative genre that will achieve recovery by itself, not without developing an effective public health system, without adequate professional practices and without balanced and fair societies for all citizens, whether they suffer from a mental disorder or not.

Acknowledgements

This work was carried out within the framework of the research project funded by the Government of Spain [PSI2016–80112–P] entitled "Challenges of the self: Identity reconstruction in situations of inequality and social exclusion".

References

Anthony, W.A. (1993). Recovery from mental illness: The guiding vision of the mental health system in the 1990s. *Innovations and Research*, 2, 17–24.

Arias-Sánchez, S., Saavedra, J., Santamaría, A., & Smorti, A. (2019). Remembering the medical practices: How health workers narrate their most negative experiences. *Memory Studies*, Online First. https://doi.org/10.1177/1750698019829864.

Bakhtin, M. (1987). *Speech genres and other late essays.* Austin: University of Texas Press.

Berlant, L. (2011). *Cruel optimism.* Durham, NC: Duke University Press.

Broyard, A (2013). *Ebrio de enfermedad* [*Intoxicated by my illness*]. Segovia: La uña rota.

Bruner, J. (1991). *Actos de significado.* Madrid: Alianza Editorial.

Bury, M. (1982). Chronic illness as biographical disruption. *Sociology of Health and Ilness*, 4(2), 167–182.

Charon, R. (2001). Narrative medicine: A model for empathy, reflection, profession and trust. *Journal of the American Medical Association*, 286(15), 1897–1902.

Costa, L., Voronka, J., Landry, D., Reid, J., McFarlane, B., Reville, D., & Church, K. (2012). Recovering our stories: A small act of resistance. *Studies in Social Justice*, 6 (1), 85–101.

Falconer, R. (2005). *Hell in contemporary literature.* Edinburgh: Edinburgh University Press.

Frank, A. (1995). *The wounded storyteller: Body, illness, and ethics.* Chicago: Chicago University Press.

The Future Vision Coalition. (2009). *A future vision of mental health.* London: The Future Vision Coalition. Retrieved from: www.newvisionformentalhealth.org.uk/A_future_vision_for_mental_health.pdf.

Gergen, K.J. & Gergen, M.M. (1986). Narrative form and the construction of psychological science. In T.R. Sarbin (Ed.), *Narrative psychology (pp.* 22–44). New York: Praeger.

Greenberg, M. (2008). *Hurry down sunshine.* New York: Other Press.

Haire, J. (2008). *Don't mind me.* London: Chipmunka Publishing.

Hart, L. (1997). *Phone at nine just to say you are alive.* London: Macmillan.

Hornbacher, M. (1999). *Wasted: A memoir of anorexia and bulimia.* London: Flamingo.

Hydén, L.C. (1997). Illness narratives. *Sociology of Health and Illness*, 19, 48–69.

Jacobson, N. & Curtis, L. (2000). Recovery as policy in mental health services: Strategies emerging from the States. *Psychiatric Rehabilitation Journal*, 23, 333–341.

Kavan, A. (1940). *Asylum pieces.* New York: Peter Owen Publishers.

Kleinman, A. (1988). *The illness narratives: Suffering, healing and the human condition.* New York: Basic Books.

Lerany, M., Bird, V., Williams, J., & Slade, M. (2011). Conceptual framework for personal recovery in mental health: Systematic review and narrative synthesis. *The British Journal of Psychiatry*, 199, 445–452. doi:10.1192/bjp.bp.110.083733.

Llewellyn-Beardsley, J., Rennick-Egglestone, S., Callard, F., Crawford, P., Farkas, M., Hui, A., Manley, D., McGranahan, R., Pollock, K., Ramsay, A., Tore Sælør, K., Wright, N., & Slade, M. (2019). Characteristics of mental health recovery narratives: Systematic review and narrative synthesis. *PLoS ONE*, 14(3), e0214678. https://doi.org/10.1371/journal.pone.0214678.

Lucius-Hoene, G. & Deppermann, A. (2002). *Rekonstruktion narrativer Identität. Ein Arbeitsbuch zur Analyse narrativer Interviews.* Opladen: Leske and Budrich.

Lysaker, P.H. & Lysaker, J. (2002). Narrative structure in psychosis schizophrenia and disruptions in the dialogical self. *Theory & Psychology*, 12, 207–220.

Lysaker, P.H., Hamm, J.A., Vohs, J., Kukla, M., Pattison, M.L., Leonhardt, B.L., & Lysaker, J.T. (2018). Understanding the course of self-disorders and alterations in self experience in schizophrenia: Implications from research on metacognition. *Current Psychiatry Reviews*, 14, 160–170.

McAdams, D.P. (2008). American identity: The redemptive self. *The General Psychologist*, 43, 20–27.

McAdams, D.P. & Bowman, P.J. (2001). Narrating life's turning points: Redemption and contamination. In D.P. McAdams, R.H. Josselson, & A. Lieblich (Eds.), *Turns in the road: Narrative studies of lives in transition (pp.* 3–34). Washington, DC: American Psychological Association.

McAdams, D.P. & McLean, K.C. (2013). Narrative identity. *Current Directions in Psychological Science*, 22(3), 233–238.

North, C. (1990). *Welcome, silence: My triumph over schizophrenia*. London: Arrow Books.

Price-Robertson, R., Manderson, L., & Duff, C. (2017). Mental ill health, recovery and the family assemblage. *Culture, Medicine, and Psychiatry*, 41(3), 407–430. https://doi.org/10.1007/s11013-017-9522-2.

Price-Robertson, R., Obradovic, A., & Morgan, B. (2016). Relational recovery: Beyond individualism in the recovery approach. *Advances in Mental Health*, 15(2), 108–120. doi:10.1080/18387357.2016.1243014.

Rennick-Egglestone, S., Ramsay, A., McGranahan, R., Llewellyn-Beardsley, J., Hui, A., Pollock, K., Repper, J., Yeo, C., Ng, F., Roe, J., Gillard, S., Thornicroft, G., Booth, S., & Slade, M. (2019). The impact of mental health recovery narratives on recipients experiencing mental health problems: Qualitative analysis and change model. *PLoS ONE*, 14(12), e0226201. https://doi.org/10.1371/journal.pone.0226201.

Ricoeur, P. (1987). *Tiempo y narración*. Madrid: Cristiandad.

Robinson, I. (1990). Personal narratives, social careers and medical courses: Analysing life trajectories in autobiographies of people with multiple sclerosis. *Social Science and Medicine*, 30, 1173–1186.

Saavedra, L. (2009a). Schizophrenia, narrative and change: Andalusian care homes as novel sociocultural context. *Culture, Medicine and Psychiatry*, 33, 163–184.

Saavedra, J. (2009b). How can we approach to traumatic stories in psychosocial rehabilitation contexts? A case study of a patient of paranoid schizophrenia. *Salud Colectiva*, 5(2), 225–235.

Saavedra, J. (2011). How to find a place in the world: Exploring people's experiences recovering from serious mental disorders. *Ciências, Saúde – Manguinhos*, 18, 121–139.

Saavedra, J., Cubero, M., & Crawford, P. (2009). Incomprehensibility in the narratives of individuals with a diagnosis of schizophrenia. *Qualitative Health Research*, 19, 1548–1558.

Saavedra, J., López, M., González, S., & Cubero, R. (2016). Does employment promote recovery? Meanings from work experience in people diagnosed with serious mental illness. *Culture, Medicine and Psychiatry*, 40(3), 507–532. doi:10.1007/s11013-015-9481-4.

Saavedra, J. & Vélez, N. (2011). The other self: Psychopathology and literature. *Medical Humanities*, 32, 257–267.

Sacks, O. (1985). *The man who mistook his wife for a hat*. New York: Basic Books.

Schacter, D.L., & Addis, D.R. (2007). The cognitive neuroscience of constructive memory: Remembering the past and imagining the future. *Philosophical Transactions of the Royal Society of London*, 362, 773–786.

Slade, M. & Longden, E. (2015). Empirical evidence about recovery and mental health. *BMC Psychiatry*, 15(285), 2–14.

Slade, M., Leamy, M., Bacon, F., Janosik, M., Le Boutillier, C., Williams, J., & Bird, V. (2012). International differences in understanding recovery: Systematic review. *Epidemiology and Psychiatric Sciences*, 21, 353–364.

Voronka, J. (2016). The politics of "people with Lived Experience": Experiential authority and the risks of strategic essentialism. *Philosophy, Psychiatry, and Psychology*, 23(3), 189–201. https://doi.org/10.1353/ppp.2016.0017.

Woods, A., Hart, A., & Spandler, H. (2019). The recovery narratives: Politics and possibilities of a genre. *Culture, Psychiatry and Medicine*, Online First.

7 (Re)constructing identity after aphasia

A preliminary study about how people with aphasia describe their selves

Sara Yuste, Andrés Santamaría, Mercedes Cubero and Manuel L. de la Mata

While literature on the impact of aphasia on the quality of life of the patient, his/her caregivers and families, his/her employment, etc., is abundant, there is a lack of data concerning identity construction of the patient after aphasia. This chapter focuses on the analysis of the identity of people with aphasia, based on the responses to the question "Who am I?" posed by the Twenty Statement Test (TST). More specifically, we have analysed the characteristics of self-descriptions about different stages of life – before damage, after damage, and in the future of people suffering from aphasia – considering brain damage (stroke) as a turning point in their lives.

Human beings are storytelling animals. In this sense, people construct stories about themselves and about others to make sense of their personal and social experiences. This suggests that stories are specific to human nature (Bruner, 1997). So, people are continuously constructing an integrative story for life. In other words, they construct a narrative identity. Narrative identity can be understood as the story of the self that interweaves the reconstructed past, the current present, and the projected future, developing a sense of unity and meaning – sense of self – in the individual (McAdams & McLean, 2013). These narratives of personal experiences are dynamic reflections about how people recall their experiences, as well as subjective constructions that have objective impacts. However, in order to construct an integrative and coherent story for life, we need to develop a description of our self, and in order to do that, language and narrative are crucial.

Language is the mediating tool through which we construct and express our identities. We are, in many ways, our language, our self-narratives. The meaning of who we are is always a linguistic and narrative construction. We are words, we define ourselves with words, and when words are missing, our possibilities as human beings are limited and our concept of ourselves is affected. So, what happens when someone's ability to narrate is reduced? What happens with their identity when people become unable to use their words? These questions are crucial for people living with aphasia, since their language is severely impaired suddenly, possibly evoking an identity crisis (Shadden, 2005). Language impairment dramatically impacts the person's quality of life in many areas, including interpersonal relationships, the ability or capacity to work, the ability to construct a strong sense of self, perceived self-efficacy, autonomy, etc. It means a disruption of the sense of self, of altered roles and relationships. According to sociocultural theories, identity is created by generating life narratives through interaction with others (McAdams, 2003). In this sense, in social construction-oriented theories, identity is equal to narrative identity. This impact of aphasia on identity is frequently acknowledged, but only a few studies have focused on self-narratives as a tool for understanding and researching this linguistic and communicative disability and its relationship with the self-making process in people with aphasia. So, when the individual's linguistic, communicative, and narrative abilities are impaired by aphasia, the individual suffers a loss of identity. Thus, to understand aphasia, we need to explore how the lives and selves of people with aphasia are constructed and shaped by language and discourse, not only at an individual level but also at a social (communicative) level.

Therefore, the aim of this chapter is to analyse the self-descriptions of people with aphasia in different stages of their lives, considering brain damage as a turning point. The study focuses on the analysis of the identity (re)construction processes in people with acquired brain damage which resulted in different types of aphasia. More specifically, we are interested in analysing how people suffering from aphasia due to brain damage describe their self at different times in their lives – before and after the onset of aphasia and their projection into the future – using a reduced version of the TST. Unfortunately, for a patient with aphasia, "Who am I now?" often does not correspond with "Who was I?" before the disorder (Mackay, 2003), and beyond, with
"Who will I be?" in the future.

Some brief notes on aphasia disorder

Traditionally, aphasia has been considered an alteration in the ability to use language, which implies a deficit in verbal communication resulting from brain damage. In this way, we can consider aphasia as a communication disorder resulting from injury to the language areas of brain, causing impairments and disorders in the ability to produce (anomie and paraphasia) and comprehend language (Ali & Anwar, 2019). Research in this field shows that the most common cause of aphasia is cerebrovascular accidents (brain stroke), causing almost 85% of all cases (Maas et al., 2012).

Establishing a typology for aphasia is not an easy task. Different classifications with diverse nomenclatures have been proposed. One of the main difficulties in developing a common framework in the field is scholars' diversity of theoretical and methodological perspectives. One of the most common aphasia disorders is expressive aphasia, or the inability to fluently produce and express spoken or written language (Behrns, Ahlsén, & Wengelin, 2010; Guina & Guina, 2018). In other types of aphasia, patients may have impaired language comprehension, and in others, there are both problems of production and comprehension (Ali & Anwar, 2019).

Therefore, aphasia is a language disability caused by brain injury (usually a stroke). Depending on different factors (brain location, severity of the stroke, and time since the onset), the linguistic consequences may vary (Pedersen, Vinter, & Olsen, 2004).

However, beyond these linguistic impairments, one of the most characteristic aspects of aphasia is reduced capacity to communicate. People with aphasia face profound social dysfunction in their lives (Lyon & Shadden, 2001). One of the greatest losses is the reduction of the communicative fluency and flexibility required to face the complex challenges involved in everyday social interactions (Shadden & Agan, 2004). This makes daily activities very difficult. And that is not the only loss. Aphasia is not simply related to language and communication. Recently, socio-pragmatic approaches that address the communicative resources and social consequences of aphasia have emerged (Duchan & Byng, 2004). In this vein, it is necessary to consider another aspect that, although less addressed by researchers, has special relevance and is closely connected with language and communication: identity. As Ali and Anwar (2019) point out, people with aphasia do not only suffer a brain infarction, but an ego infarction as well. For them, the injury also has an influence on the "self" of the patient (Shadden & Agan, 2004), which contributes to the damage in identity (Shadden, 2005). Although many studies in the field of aphasiology have focused on the analysis of the diverse consequences of aphasia disorder, only a few have examined the effects of aphasia on patients' selves. That is, on their identity(ies).

Communication, language, and identity in people with aphasia: aphasia as an identity challenge

As we know, individuals are able to transmit or receive information through language, both oral and written, and with that each individual develops his or her own image. The image that we create of ourselves and that we express to others constitutes the support of personal identity within a group. As social beings, human beings need communication to construct their identities, both individually and collectively, within society. Throughout our lives, we are surrounded by acts that allow us to develop our own identity. These events are mediated by communication. As Ali and Anwar (2019) point out, we project our identities onto others during social interactions through communication, and others approve or disapprove this identity. But what happens when a person suffers from aphasia? Is his or her identity changed by these communicative limitations? Does suffering from this disorder make identity change? When a social interaction and the subsequent discourse produced present a negative sense of one's self, the identity and self-respect of the subject suffers. This happens in aphasia disorders. All of us need a strong and stable sense of identity to achieve a state of well-being and improve our quality of life. Aphasia patients present great difficulties in developing this sense of identity, so their well-being and quality of life are damaged. In this sense, and in relation to the close link between language and the construction of a personal identity, in our opinion, the study of aphasia can be considered as a context of special relevance for studying the identity (re)construction process.

But what is the notion of identity that we adopt? Our notion of identity has been extensively developed in Chapter 2 of this volume, so we will be very brief here in its conceptualization.

Identity (and self) has been understood in numerous ways in the literature. In this sense, there are authors that use the terms "personal identity" and "self" as synonyms, and others, as different notions. We will not enter this exciting debate, and we will use both terms – identity and self – interchangeably, even while being aware of the nuances involved.

In this vein, our view of personal identity is not that of a homogeneous and stable entity, but quite the opposite. The self takes meaning depending on the historical circumstances of the culture in which it participates (Bruner, 1997). Identity – self – will be understood not as a given, pre-existing, and static entity, but as built throughout life (de la Mata, Santamaría, Hansen, & Ruiz, 2015; de la Mata, Santamaría, & Ruiz, 2016). We adopt a constructivist, discursive, social, and cultural view of identity, in which this phenomenon is regarded as a multiple and continuously negotiated reality. Identity is understood as a process by which individuals, through the social and cultural practices in which they are involved, discursively establish who they are in their relationship with other individuals and with social contexts and settings. In other words, identity is the result of what people do and say in their daily practices, not a monolithic or purely psychological concept.

Over the last twenty years, research has shown that the construction of identity can be achieved through narration. For example, Schiffrin (1996) conceives narrative as a linguistic lens through which to discover people's own (somewhat idealized) views of themselves as situated in a social structure. De Fina, Schiffrin, and Bamberg (2006) stress that, through narration, people enact and negotiate personal and social roles, relationships, and their membership in a specific community. A similar view is put forth by Schrauf (2000, p. 128), who argues that "personal and social identities are proffered, contested and negotiated in discursive practices". However, it does not imply that the individual rejects continuity and coherence in the narration of himself/herself. Identity thus implies, at the same time:

a a conscious feeling of personal uniqueness (I am unique and different from others);
b a sense of permanence and continuity over time (I am the same person as in my youth);
c that which unites us with other people and leads us to share with them a series of characteristics (I am a woman).

The study: how people with aphasia describe their selves in different stages of their lives

In this study, we focus on the analysis of how patients with aphasia describe themselves at different times in their lives: before the stroke causing aphasia, after the stroke, and how they project their self into the future. The study of how the self develops has focused on the descriptions that people make of themselves at the present time (current self). However, not many studies have focused on analysing the nature and function of those descriptions about their past and, especially, projections of the self in the future – possible selves (Markus & Nurius, 1986). This is related to the ideal selves that we would like to become, but also to those we could become, and even those we are afraid of becoming. In this study, the following research questions are asked:

- How are self-descriptions of people with aphasia characterized?
- Are these self-descriptions maintained or changed throughout three time periods: before the stroke causing aphasia, after the stroke, and in their projection into the future?

In order to answer these research questions, the following objectives were formulated:

- To explore identity (re)construction of the patients with aphasia after an episode of a stroke.
- To identify the main characteristics of their self-descriptions constitutive of their identity.
- To study the possible changes in the self-descriptions of these patients before the stroke causing aphasia, after the stroke, and in their projection into the future.

Method

The study was based on a cross-sectional analytical strategy, in which the self-descriptions of the participants about different stages in relation to the episode of brain damage (before the stroke causing aphasia, after the episode, and in their future self-projection) were compared. The response variable was identity, measured through the participants' self-descriptions collected and analysed with a category system that included three dimensions (organization of the self-descriptions, the plane of the self-descriptions, and thematic reference).

The study of self-descriptions has employed different methodologies. We applied an open-ended approach to the analysis of TST responses. TST has been widely used for more than five decades to explore how individuals think and speak about themselves, using their own words.

Participants

The participants in this study were four subjects: two women and two men, aged 45–69. All of them had suffered brain damage and consequently aphasia. The participants were selected among those who maintained a communicative level that allowed them to participate in this study. Most of them suffered from anomic residual aphasia, having greater limitations in understanding the concepts. The participants selected could carry out the tasks required without major problems. Tables 7.1 and 7.2 provide a detailed explanation of the characteristics of the participants.

All participants were receiving or had received language rehabilitation therapy.

They were contacted through the Association for the Prevention and Rehabilitation of Aphasia (ARPA) in Seville. Participation was voluntary, unpaid, and based on informed consent.

Table 7.1 Socio-demographic characteristics of group members with aphasia

Name	*Sex*	*Age*	*Educational level*	*Marital status*	*Number of children*	*Work activity*
IG	Female	47	High	Married	2	Billing and treasury manager
RU	Male	69	Low	Married	3	Fruit seller
VI	Male	67	High	Married	4	Architect and engineer
SV	Female	45	High	Divorced	2	Teacher and city councillor

Table 7.2 Characteristics of group members with aphasia about aphasia

Name	*Age at stroke*	*Current severity of damage*	*Associated diagnosis*
IG	42	Low	Comprehension deficit.Anomie.
RU	64	Severe	Problems in understanding concepts, lack of fluency, and grammatical difficulty.
VI	63	Medium	Deficit in auditory discrimination.Deficits in the construction of words.
SV	45	Low	Unable to pronounce complex words. Anomie and dysprosody.

Instruments

The TST technique is highly valued as an instrument to assess spontaneous self-concepts and how these concepts vary depending on social and cultural factors (Santamaría, de la Mata, Hansen, & Ruiz, 2010). The literature in this field has traditionally considered two dimensions of the self: (a) *personal* aspects of the self that differentiate the self from others; and (b) *social* aspects of the self that reflect his or her relationship with others (Sedikides & Brewer, 2001). The latter has been divided into a relational and a collective level. As some authors point out (Santamaría et al., 2010), the TST is an instrument that contrasts with psychometric instruments and standardized questionnaires that use Likert-type scales. The TST provides a more qualitative and exploratory approach to categorization of relevant meanings associated with participants' self-descriptions. For that reason, it was used in this study. In this test, the participants are asked to complete 20 sentences beginning with "I am", with any words, phrases, or sentences that the participants feel describe them the best. In our study, we used a reduced version of this test, with only ten sentences to be completed. This is in accordance with previous studies (Santamaría et al., 2010; Wang, 2001), given the difficulty with which participants completed the 20 sentences. In this modified version, participants also had to generate self-descriptions for their possible selves, i.e. as projected into the future (Markus & Nurius, 1986). These possible selves are the projections of the self in the following years. The analysis of the open answers (self-descriptions) requires the use of a category system. In our case, three dimensions of analysis were considered.

Procedure

The questionnaires were applied to all study participants individually, in the therapy rooms of the Asociación Ayuda Afasia (Spain's equivalent to the National Aphasia Association) in Madrid, and in one case in the participant's home. The instructions were the same for all subjects. Before completing the TST, each participant signed the informed consent form. After each participant read and understood the instructions, they were asked to complete the sentences referring to the three stages ("I was …" for the past, "I am …" for the present, and "I will be …" for the future). The average time to complete the three versions was 30 minutes.

Coding

After reviewing previous studies, a category system was developed by the authors. In this category system, three different analysis dimensions of the self-descriptions were considered: organization, self plane, and thematic reference (see Table 7.3).

Table 7.3 System of categories

Dimension	*Dimension definitions*	*Category*	*Category definitions*	*Examples*
		Personal (PER)	Descriptions refer to PER+ “I will be brave” qualities, attitudes, or PERS-: “I was physical and psychological insecure” attributes of themselves.	
The organization of self-description	Categories referring to the relationship of the subject with his/her social context	Relational (REL)	The participant describes therself through his or her relationships with others.	“I was calm with my students” “I am good with my son”
		Group (GRO)	The participant is described through their identification with a group (by occupation, place of origin, sex, sexual orientation, etc.).	“I belonged to a tennis club” “I will be a triathlete
		Description (DES)	Descriptions refer to physical or socio-demographic characteristics of him or herself.	“I was brown” “My name is Javier”
The self plane	Categories referring to what the subject currently does or how they are.	Action (ACT)	Descriptions refer to the participant as performing or being involved in actions.	“I travelled” “I cook”
		Reflection (REF)	Descriptions reflect on his or her way of being, life, or problems.	“I was too nervous” “I will be happier”

(Continued)

Table 7.3 (Cont.)

Dimension	*Dimension definitions*	*Category*	*Category definitions*	*Examples*
Thematic reference	Categories referring to the type of content that the subject is talking about.	Bio-psycho-social references (BPS)	Descriptions refer to physical, psychological, and social characteristics of the participants.	"I am Italian" "I will be thinner"
		Relational references (REL)	Descriptions refer to people with whom they have close ties (family, friends, coworkers, etc.).	"I loved my children" "I am a good mother"
		Work or training activities references (FOR)	Descriptions refer to work or training activities.	"I was a plumber" "I love my job very much"
		Leisure activities references (LEI)	Descriptions refer to extracurricular activities that have to do with personal preferences.	"I like football" "I will do a triathlon"

Two observers trained in the category system coded the self-description. Reliability was calculated using the Kappa index. Kappa values were 0.89, 0.92, and 0.90 for the three dimensions respectively. The Global Kappa index was 0.98.

Results and discussion

This section will be structured based on the presentation of the aspects that characterize each of the participants according to the time to which the self-descriptions refer and in relation to the three dimensions of analysis established in the category system. Due to the nature of the study, no statistical analysis was carried out. A comparative table of the results in relation to each of the dimensions is presented in Table 7.4.

In order to have an overview of the data, the following table shows the category or categories that collect 50% or more of the self-descriptions given by the four participants in the study, in each dimension and in each of the three stages studied (Table 7.4). Next, the results obtained in each of the cases will be described.

As can be seen in Table 7.4, generally, there does not seem to be a marked difference in the descriptions made by the four participants. Thus, in the "organization of self-description" dimension, positive descriptions predominated in qualities, attitudes, and physical or psychological attributes about themselves. At present, negative self-descriptions predominated only in one participant – precisely the one who currently has the most severe brain damage. In "the self plane" dimension, reflective self-descriptions predominated. However, it was at present when, in two cases, participants described themselves favourably in relation to performing or being involved in actions. As for the third dimension, "thematic reference", the majority of the participants' self-description referred to physical, psychological, and social characteristics.

Notwithstanding that, these results can be misleading without a detailed analysis of each individual case.

If we focus on the first case, IG, the most relevant fact in the first dimension is that, in the descriptions about how she was before aphasia, there were no positive self-descriptions; she described herself in a negative way (PER- = 50%) with expressions like "very strict about work" or "worried about what others would say". She only described herself positively through her relationships with others ("good wife" or "good mother") (REL = 46%). However, at present, all her descriptions were personal and positive ("I see myself living life with enthusiasm") and in the future these exceeded 80% ("I will laugh at myself" or "I will be a reference for improvement in my environment"). Based on the above, we can infer that IG's aphasia was a turning point in her self-concept and also happened in an unexpected direction. It seems as if having overcome the traumatic event of suffering aphasia has made her have a more positive vision of herself. If, as proposed by Oyserman and collaborators (Oyserman, Bybee, & Terry, 2006; Oyserman & Fryberg, 2006), the potential

Table 7.4 Summary of the results of the four cases in each dimension in the present, past, and future

	The organization of self-description			*The self plane*			*Thematic reference*		
	Past	*Present*	*Future*	*Past*	*Present*	*Future*	*Past*	*Present*	*Future*
IG		PER+	PER+	REF	ACT	REF		BPSO	BPSO
									REL
RU	PER+	PER-	PER+	REF	REF	REF	BPSO	BPSO	BPSO
VI	PER+	PER+	PER+	REF	REF	REF	BPSO	BPSO	BPSO
SV	PER+		PER+	REF	REF	REF	BPSO	BPSO	BPSO

or future selves can have a motivating power for action – "roadmaps" – in this case it seems clear that she has high expectations about her future in the medium and long term.

In the second dimension of analysis, the self plane, both in the present and in the future, 100% of the descriptions of the self were of a reflective nature. However, in the present, these descriptions decreased (REF = 40%) and most of the descriptions were of herself performing or being involved in actions (60%), which supports the theory of aphasia being a reconstruction of identity for IG (in terms of Shadden, 2005). As we argued previously, identity is understood not as a given, pre-existing, and static entity, but as the result of what people do and say in their daily practices (de la Mata et al., 2015, 2016). These changes in identity also require reflective processes (Bruner, 2003; McAdams, 2003) about what the individuals were like, what aspirations or interests they had, and what they want or hope to be in the future. These individuals take as a reference point what they are and what abilities they have at present ("I was not calm" or "I will not care about what others say"). Perhaps that is precisely why there is less reflection and more description about what actions they can carry out in the present, as opposed to those they could do just after suffering brain damage ("Now I can read"). We believe that the fact that IG, like all the other cases, undergoes rehabilitation therapy makes it easier for her to focus on the present in descriptions about her potential. Therefore, in the self plane, descriptions of actions such as "I am active" or "Now I can talk" abounded.

In the thematic reference, as in the previous dimension, IG shows a similar pattern in the past and in the future. In both times, those descriptions referring to physical, psychological, and social characteristics of the participants were distributed equally, as were the descriptions referring to people with whom they have close ties (BPSO and REL = 46% in the past and 50% in the future). In the present, however, descriptions referring to bio-psychosocial characteristics increased (BPSO = 80%) and those referring to relational characteristics decreased (REL = 20%).

From what we have seen, we can conclude that aphasia has meant an identity change for IG. In the past, she had a negative view of herself ("I was boring before") and she was more focused on her work and less sensitive and involved with her environment. After suffering brain damage and after her work in therapeutic rehabilitation, she sees herself as a stronger and more courageous woman, capable of achieving the goals she sets out, which she expresses with everything she is capable of today and what she could not do immediately after suffering brain damage. Perhaps because of this analysis of her achievements and her current low damage, she maintains this attitude in her possible selves, and it can drive her to take future actions that are consistent with an outlook of herself that she sees as "happy" and "calm".

In the second case, RU, negative personal descriptions are concentrated in the present (PER- = 50%) in the dimension of the organization of self-description, with expressions like "I'm dumb" or "I'm depressed". This is not surprising, as RU is the participant with most severe brain damage at present. This makes him quite dependent on his environment, which is perhaps the reason for the existence of relational descriptions only in the present (REL = 35%). However, this negative assessment of his present condition does not seem to affect his view of himself either in the past (PER+ = 80%) or in the future (PER+ = 75%) – perhaps precisely because of his current assessment. As we mentioned in IG's case, the reference point is always the present, and this is seen as so negative that he may idealize both his past and his future with expressions such as "I was cheerful" or "I will be better".

In relation to the self plane, we observed that both in the past and present, 100% of his descriptions were reflective in nature. Perhaps this constant comparison between what he was and what he is now, after the stroke, justifies this evaluative nature. However, although his descriptions of his possible selves maintain a high level of reflection (REF = 50%), they include aspects related to actions that he hoped to be able to carry out (ACT = 40%) ("I'll understand more").

In relation to the thematic reference dimension, in the past (BPSO = 100%), present (BPSO = 67%), and future (BPSO = 75%), RU focuses his descriptions on themes related to psychological characteristics, such as "I was cheerful", "I am pessimistic", or "I would like to be happier". But, perhaps most interestingly, there are themes related to his relationship with others (REL = 17%), which is not surprising given his high level of dependency. It is also interesting that topics related to training appear (FOR = 17% in the present and FOR = 25% in the future), since this participant has a very low educational level ("I will study more things").

Thus, RU's descriptions about himself show us, in the past, a very positive self-concept, as he saw himself as someone "happy" and "independent". After the stroke and the serious sequels he suffers today, he perceives himself as a less capable person, with many limitations and, therefore, more dependent on his environment. In the future, however, he seems to increase his confidence in his own abilities and describes himself through his actions, which in many cases are related to his own training ("I will study more things"). We believe that the desire to overcome his present is what makes him construct a more positive outlook of himself in the future. Like IG, we believe that this has a lot to do with the very therapy in which they are involved. It does not only work in the area of neurocognitive rehabilitation, but also deals with social-emotional aspects. From this perspective, we emphasize the role of narrative therapy in the construction of new selves, in the sense that de Fina et al. (2006) or Schrauf (2000) argued when proposing that personal and social identity is constructed in discursive practices and through narratives.

In the third case, VI, positive personal descriptions predominated in the three times considered in the first dimension, although they represented 100% of the uttered statements in the future, 83% in the past, and 60% in the present. In this case, it is worth mentioning the existence in the past (PER- = 17%) and in the present (PER- = 10%) of some negative personal descriptions such as "I was very stressed" and "sometimes I am sad and have low morale". It is especially interesting how, in the present, VI described himself through his identification with a group by his occupation or his place of origin (GRO = 30%), such as when he describes himself as "I am an engineer" or "I am Italian". In this case, although perhaps in a less evident way than in the previous ones, it seems that the projection of his selves in the future was more positive.

At the self plane, the reflective nature of his descriptions continues to predominate in the past (REF = 100%), present (REF = 70%), and future (REF = 88%). However, in this case, the descriptions through actions were replaced by descriptions that mention an "I" that is presented in relation to physical and socio-demographic characteristics (DES = 30% in the present and DES = 22% in the future). These reflections on what he was, is, and will be, on his past, present, and future interests, desires, and worries, are his own self-narratives. This is the sense in which McAdams and McLean (2013) speak of identity as a narrative construction of personal experiences, as the story of the self that reconstructed past, the current present, and the projected future. Thus, the narrative woven from therapy and what they internalize and elaborate about their autobiographical experiences represents who they are and how they define their selves.

In the thematic reference, descriptions of bio-psychosocial content are those that predominated in the three times, especially in the future (BPSO = 100%, in the past BPSO = 83% and in the present BPSO = 80%). In the past, they were mixed with descriptions that have to do with leisure; and in the present, with those related to studies or work. It is interesting how descriptions of him involved in leisure activities such as "I travelled a lot" only appeared in the past.

In the past, VI described himself as being active and involved in his work, which made him stressed out and withdrawn from relationships. In the present, however, he sees himself as a calmer person and alludes to more emotional qualities: "I am more loving". In the future, there is a considerable increase in positive descriptions: "I will be more cheerful and more reflective". It seems as if the damage has made him appreciate the small moments in life and the support of his family, and minimize the importance of his work environment in his life.

In the fourth and last case, SV, positive self-descriptions predominated both in the past (PER+ = 72%) and in the future (PER+ = 72%), as shown in RU and VI. Negative self-descriptions, however, were mainly concentrated in the present (PER- = 17%), as in RU, because although the sequels of SV's stroke have not been very serious at present, she described herself as having fewer skills than in the past, especially those related to work aspects: "I am more negative about my achievements". At present, however, she describes herself as more interactive with her environment, especially with her family: "I am a better mother because I am more present" (REL = 17%).

In the second dimension, the pattern found in other cases continues. The majority of descriptions of the self are reflexive in the three times, although there is a decrease in the present (REF = 66%) with respect to the past (REF = 72%) and the future (REF = 100%). Similarly, the present concentrated all the descriptions of the self, with SV defining herself as being involved or carrying out actions (ACT = 17%) always in relation to what the stroke hindered ("now I can run"). As we have already stated when describing other cases, the aphasia produced by a cerebrovascular accident marks a turning point (before and after) in autobiographical narratives, introducing, therefore, changes in their descriptions of identity. These changes are necessary to give continuity, integration, and meaning to an identity that has been "interrupted" or "destabilized" by the transformations in physical, psychological, and social abilities that brain damage has brought about (Shadden, 2005).

In the thematic reference, descriptions of the self were mostly bio-psycho-social, although they progressively decreased from the past (BPSO = 77%) to the present (BPSO = 66%) and the future (BPSO = 58%). An interesting fact is the emergence of leisure-related descriptions in the future (LEI = 28%).

Thus, SV described herself in the past in a positive way, but such descriptions were preferably related to her profession: "I was very active", "I was political". In the future, however, such positive descriptions of herself were related to leisure activities. In this sense, again, the present can be considered as a turning point (McAdams, 2003). The perception of herself, her identity, has thus changed after suffering the consequences of brain damage. Aphasia seems to have changed her life preferences and directed them towards herself and her family.

To conclude, despite their limitations, our results allow us to establish certain general guidelines. In this sense, we find that in all the cases the descriptions have been personal, that is, they identify and distinguish themselves from others, among other things by attributes that we might call "characterological"; by their "lifestyle" reflected mainly in their consumption habits; by their personal network of "intimate relationships" (alter ego); by the set of "valuable objects" they possess; and by their untiring personal biography. These results are those obtained in most of the studies carried out with people in Western countries. It can be observed that, within these personal descriptions, positive descriptions decrease considerably when it comes to the present time, in comparison with the past and the future.

On the other hand, as has been seen in this study, all participants describe themselves in the past (before the injury) in a positive way when it comes to purely intellectual and physical abilities, while many participants allude to negative characteristics that they saw in themselves before, and now, thanks to the new outlook they have of themselves due to the injury, those negative characteristics have disappeared. We are referring to the fact that suffering a setback of this nature makes them appreciate other facets of their day-to-day life, which went unnoticed previously. It is at the present time (after the injury) that negative descriptions appear in most cases (especially at the level of intellect and cognitive resources). However, in spite of seeing their diminished faculties, they draw a positive outlook. All of them see a glimmer of improvement, they see themselves in the future in a more positive way, with the capacity to overcome. Most are confident that they will be better in the future. In a way, we could say they are resilient.

The fact of suffering a life impact thus marks a turning point in the construction of one's identity, as well as in the possible negotiation of new identities after the damage. Thus, in the case of aphasia, a strong sense of identity will be associated with well-being and with a better quality of life (Cooney, Murphy, & O'Shea 2009).

Concluding remarks

The present study examined the process of identity (re)construction, in terms of self-descriptions of people with aphasia. More specifically, it focused on the analysis of the differences in these descriptions in three dimensions of analysis (organization of the descriptions, the self plane, and thematic reference). In this sense, we have compared the categories of self-description in three different stages of life (before the brain damage that caused aphasia, at the present time after the damage, and the projection of their selves into the future).

To conclude, and after the analysis of the four cases studied, as well as the outlook that each of them has given regarding their identity in the three time periods considered, there are factors worth highlighting. First, the importance of language and communication for the integrity of the individual in society; that is, in establishing a strong sense of identity. When linguistic and communicative abilities are impaired by aphasia, the individual suffers a loss of his or her identity, of the identity s/he has built in society so far. Shadden (2005) describes this loss or diminishment of the sense of self that is associated with the onset of aphasia as "identity theft". For her, aphasia can be considered as a "hazard to identity". Additionally, the study has enabled us to verify how people who have suffered from brain damage causing aphasia reconstruct their identity, and how they recreate their world and their selves to reconfigure the aspect of that identity modified/affected by brain damage. Somehow, they re-negotiate a strong and positive identity after the vital changes associated with the onset of aphasia. But how can they do it? Perhaps, as Simmons-Mackie and Elman (2011) remind us, one way is to develop social connections that are coherent with a positive and robust sense of the self. Or, as Howe (2017) highlights, finding new opportunities for social participation. For all this, language and communication skills are crucial. As we have pointed out throughout the chapter, we are words, we define ourselves with words and, when words are absent, limiting our potential as human beings, the concept we have of ourselves is diminished. Others identify us with words, with language. We are our name, we are students, journalists, blonde, brown, tall, good at playing football, etc. We are totally surrounded by terms and concepts that define, identify, support, and sometimes even persecute us.

We live in a world of verbal labels, and we spend years trying to adjust to the canons of those labels, to that social norm that tells us who we are and how we are. In the case of these people, after suffering brain damage, their sense of identity (their self) is diminished in an instant. All those labels that were acquired over the years are now being diluted. With aphasia, they cannot communicate; in many cases they cannot even say their own name or identify who they are.

This study has made us wonder if they are still the same people, if they continue to maintain their same identity or the same outlook of identity that they had. We wonder if they have to reconstruct their identity, if new identities are now being forged, with these being other possible selves that facilitate their recovery and the recovery of their identity.

In our opinion, perhaps what is happening is that they are developing other "possible identities", other "possible selves" that can help facilitate their recovery. Somehow, they are initiating a negotiation process of a new identity (Shadden, 2005; Shadden & Agan, 2004; Simmons-Mackie & Elman, 2011).

Taking into account previous studies, we have confirmed the existence of a lack of studies on the vital importance that the loss of language, communication, and social connection has in the processes of (re)construction and (re)negotiation of identity. We consider it of crucial importance to continue in this line of research to facilitate the efficacy of therapies and the global and unified understanding of each patient from a clinical point of view (Musser, Wilkinson, Gilbert, & Bokhour, 2015; Shadden, 2005; Shadden & Agan, 2004; Simmons-Mackie & Elman, 2011).

Finally, this study has made us consider possible research routes that go beyond the analysis of the descriptions that people with aphasia can make of themselves, and focus our interest on the analysis of autobiographical narratives and life stories of these people – before and after the damage – that can give us clues in the study of the inextricable relationship between aphasia and identity. These studies would take into account other variables, such as the time elapsed since the damage, the support received, the available resources (both economic and social), etc. The past, present, and future are linked to one another to form a coherent plot, which provides life with unity, purpose, and meaning. This is crucial to mental health and quality of life (Corsten, Schimpf, Konradi, Keilmann, & Hardering, 2015). Based on this idea, narrative identity plays a key role. In this vein, the extent to which people restore their sense of identity and bring renewed meaning to their lives is crucial too (Clarke & Black, 2005). Life narratives facilitate the process of sense-making of the illness experience, the reconstruction of meaning and purposes of life, and the review of one's own strengths and resources that might help to overcome personal and environmental challenges (Corsten et al., 2015). This research suggests that telling stories of the self may be an important rehabilitation tool. It can be useful for clinicians when working with such interventions (Taubner, Hallén, & Wengelin, 2020).

With these data, in our opinion, perhaps we can go deeper into the relationship between linguistic and communicative difficulties associated with brain damage and aphasia, and the (re)construction of the identity of these people. As Shadden (2005) eloquently reminds us, to understand aphasia, it is critical to explore how the identity of persons with aphasia are shaped by language, discourse, and narratives.

Acknowledgements

This chapter was written with the support of the research project funded by the Government of Spain [PSI2016–80112–P] entitled "Challenges of the self: Identity reconstruction in situations of inequality and social exclusion".

References

Ali, N. & Anwar, N. (2019). Vicissitudes of aphasic identity: Discourse analysis under James Paul Gee's identity framework. *International Journal of English Linguistics*, 9, 97–110. https://doi.org/10.5539/ijel.v9n1p97.

Behrns, I., Ahlsén, E., & Wengelin, A. (2010). Aphasia and text writing. *International Journal of Language & Communication Disorders*, 45, 230–243. http://dx.doi.org/10.1080/02687930802436892.

Bruner, J. (1997). A narrative model of self construction. In J.T. Snodgrass (Ed.), *The self across psychology* (pp. 145–161). New York: New York Academy of Science.

Bruner, J. (2003). Self-making narratives. In R. Fivush & C.A. Haden (Eds.), *Autobiographical memory and the construction of a narrative self: Developmental and cultural perspectives* (pp. 209–225). Mahwah: Lawrence Erlbaum Associates Publishers.

Clarke, P. & Black, S.E. (2005). Quality of life following stroke: Negotiating disability, identity, and resources. *Journal of Applied Gerontology*, 24, 319–336. https://doi.org/10.1177%2F0733464805277976.

Cooney, A., Murphy, K., & O'Shea, E. (2009). Resident perspectives of the determinants of quality of life in residential care in Ireland. *Journal of Advanced Nursing*, 65, 1029–1038.

Corsten, S., Schimpf, E.J., Konradi, J., Keilmann, A., & Hardering, F. (2015). The participants' perspective: How biographic–narrative intervention influences identity negotiation and quality of life in aphasia. *International Journal of Language & Communication Disorders*, 50, 788–800.

de Fina, A., Schiffrin, D., & Bamberg, M. (Eds.) (2006). *Studies in interactional sociolinguistics: Vol. 23. Discourse and identity.* Cambridge: Cambridge University Press. https://doi.org/10.1017/CBO9780511584459.

De la Mata, M.L., Santamaría, A., & Ruiz, M.L. (2016). Toward the model of independence: The influence of formal schooling experience on earliest autobiographical memories and self-construals – a preliminary study. *Journal of Cross-Cultural Psychology*, 47(5), 670–679. https://psycnet.apa.org/doi/10.1177/0022022116635745.

De la Mata, M.L., Santamaría, A., Hansen, T.G.B., & Ruiz, L. (2015). Earliest autobiographical memories in college student from three countries: Towards a situated view. *Memory Studies*, 8, 151–168. https://doi.org/10.1177%2F1750698014543966.

Duchan, J.F. & Byng, S. (2004). *Challenging aphasia therapies: Broadening the discourse and extending the boundaries.* London: Psychology Press.

Guina, J. & Guina, C. (2018). Wants talk psychotherapy but cannot talk: EMDR for post-stroke depression with expressive aphasia. *Innovations in Clinical Neuroscience*, 15(1–2), 45–48.

Howe, T. (2017). Found opportunities for social participation: Facilitating inclusion of adults with aphasia. *Topics in Language Disorders*, 37(1), 38–51. https://doi.org/10.1097/TLD.0000000000000113.

Lyon, J.G. & Shadden, B.B. (2001). Treating life consequences of aphasia's chronicity. In R. Chapey (Ed.), *Language intervention strategies in aphasia and related neurogenic communication disorders* (4th Edition) (pp. 297–315). Philadelphia: Lippincott Williams and Wilkins.

Maas, M.B., Lev, M.H., Ay, H., Singhal, A.B., Greer, D.M., Smith, W.S., & Furie, K. L. (2012). The prognosis for aphasia in stroke. *Journal of Stroke and Cerebrovascular Diseases*, 21(5), 350–357. https://doi.org/10.1016/j.jstrokecerebrovasdis.2010.09.009.

McAdams, D.P. (2003). Identity and the life story. In R. Fivush & C.A. Haden (Eds.), *Autobiographical memory and the construction of a narrative self: Developmental and cultural perspectives* (pp. 187–207). Mahwah, NJ: Lawrence Erlbaum Associates.

McAdams, D.P. & McLean, K.C. (2013). Selves creating stories creating selves: A process model self-development. *Personality & Social Psychology Review*, 11(23), 262–278. https://doi.org/10.1177/1088868307301034.

Mackay, R. (2003). "Tell them who I was": The social construction of aphasia. *Disability & Society*, 18(6), 811–826. https://doi.org/10.1080/0968759032000119532.

Markus, H. & Nurius, P. (1986). Possible selves. *American Psychologist*, 41, 954–969.

Musser, B., Wilkinson, J., Gilbert, T., & Bokhour, B. (2015). Changes in identity after aphasic stroke: Implications for primary care. *International Journal for Family Medicine*, 1–8. https://doi.org/10.1155/2015/970345.

Oyserman, D. & Fryberg, S. (2006). The possible selves of diverse adolescents: Content and function across gender, race and national origin. In C. Dunkel & J. Kerpelman (Eds.), *Possible selves: Theory, research, and application* (pp. 17–39). New York: Nova.

Oyserman, D., Bybee, D., & Terry, K. (2006). Possible selves and academic outcomes: How and when possible selves impel action. *Journal of Personality and Social Psychology*, 91, 188–204. https://doi.org/10.1037/0022-3514.91.1.188.

Pedersen, P.M., Vinter, K., & Olsen, T.S. (2004). Aphasia after stroke: Type, severity and prognosis: The Copenhagen aphasia study. *Cerebrovascular Diseases*, 17, 35–43. http://dx.doi.org/10.1159/000073896.

Santamaría, A., de la Mata, M.L., Hansen, T.G.B., & Ruiz, L. (2010). Cultural self-construals of Mexican, Spanish and Danish college students: Beyond independent and interdependent self. *Journal of Cross-Cultural Psychology*, 41, 471–477. https://psycnet.apa.org/doi/10.1177/0022022109359694.

Schiffrin, D. (1996). Narrative as self-portrait: Sociolinguistic construction of identity. *Language in Society*, 25, 167–203. www.jstor.org/stable/4168695.

Schrauf, R.W. (2000). Narrative repair of threatened identity. *Narrative Inquiry*, 10(1), 1–19. https://doi.org/10.1075/ni.10.1.08sch.

Sedikides, C. & Brewer, M.B. (2001). Individual self, relational self, and collective self. In C. Sedikides & M.B. Brewer (Eds.), *Individual self, relational self, collective self.* Philadelphia: Psychology Press.

Shadden, B. (2005). Aphasia as identity theft: Theory and practice. *Aphasiology*, 19(3–5), 211–223. https://doi.org/10.1080/02687930444000697.

Shadden, B.B. & Agan, J.P. (2004). Renegotiation of identity: The social context of aphasia support groups. *Topics in Language Disorders*, 24(3), 174–186. https://doi.org/10.1097/00011363-200407000-00005.
Simmons-Mackie, N. & Elman, N.J. (2011). Negotiation of identity in group therapy for aphasia: The aphasia café. *International Journal of Language and Communication Disorders*, 46(3), 312–323. https://doi.org/10.3109/13682822.2010.507616.
Taubner, H., Hallén, M., & Wengelin, A. (2020). Still the same? Self identity dilemmas when living with post-stroke aphasia in a digitalised society. *Aphasiology*, *34*(3), 300–318. doi:10.1080/02687038.2019.1594151.
Wang, Q. (2001). Culture effects on adult's earliest childhood recollection and self-description: Implications for the relation between memory and self. *Journal of Personality and Social Psychology*, 81(2), 220–223.

8 Narratives and identity construction of children with developmental speech and language disorders

Kristine Jensen de López and Rena Lyons

Introduction

People create "a sense of identity both in the stories that they choose to tell and especially in the way they tell their stories" (Hiles, Čermák, & Chrz, 2017). Narratives, whether they are big life stories or small stories about an episode, always reveal the speaker's identity (Bamberg & Georgakopoulou, 2008). Today narrative inquiry, self-making narratives, and identity construction are well-established approaches for gaining better understandings of the lives of adults without disabilities. However, some decades ago Owens (2007) argued that the assumption that narrative inquiry could only be used with those who can tell their stories coherently should be challenged. In recent years we have seen an increase in research exploring identity and biographical disruption when adults experience acquired communication disabilities (Barrow, 2011; Glintborg, 2015; Shadden, 2005; Strong & Shadden, 2019). However, narrative approaches are still less commonly used to explore the lives of young children with disabilities.

In this chapter, we focus on a specific group of children with communication disabilities, namely children who grew up with developmental speech or language disorders. These disorders have no clear biological or neurological cause and can have significant impacts on academic and psychosocial domains. Given that identity is constructed through narratives, it is worth noting that these children may present with deficits in their narrative abilities and their ability to create autobiographical narratives (Tompkins & Jeffrey Farrar, 2011). Up until recently, there was little research on use of narrative inquiry to explore identity construction in children with developmental speech and language disorders. There is now some evidence to suggest that children with developmental speech and language disorders do construct multiple identities, negotiate their identities with others, and are quite aware of the stigma associated with being different (Lyons & Roulstone, 2017).

In our contribution to the current volume, we will first provide a short overview of some of Bruner's original concepts and thoughts about self-narratives and have these occur from a very early age of life. Following this we present a review of the sparse literature addressing identity and identity construction in children with developmental speech language disorders along with the methodological challenges when using narrative inquiry with these children (Lyons & Roulstone, 2018). Finally, we will present and discuss concrete examples and findings from our own ongoing research on how young Irish and Danish children with developmental speech and language disorders construe their disabilities and how they construct their identities in relation to their developmental challenges. From a developmental perspective, we also suggest methodological recommendations that may be useful for other researchers who wish to investigate identity construction in young children with communication disabilities.

Self-narratives and identity construction in children

The notion of self and identity are complex constructs and it is important to define terms such as self-concept, self-esteem, and identity. Baumeister (2005) defined self-concept as individuals' beliefs about themselves, including attributes such as being shy or talkative, while Meadows (2010, p. 65) argued that self-concept "sits inside our heads". The term self-esteem has been defined as one's perceptions or evaluations about oneself (Burden, 2008). Identity refers to how we see ourselves and also how others see us. According to sociocultural theories of identity, it is through interaction with the environment that individuals are able to develop a concept of self. Identities can be viewed as something that we do and are a social product that arise through interaction with others (Acton & Hird, 2004). People present themselves and interact in particular ways and are recognized as certain "kinds of person" (Gee, 2000). It is acknowledged that language plays a pivotal role in the identity construction process (Gee, Allen, & Clinton, 2001).

Bruner (1997) argued that self-narratives emerge from dialogue, driven by a metacognitive process, and that self-narratives are purpose-built for the specific occasion, as opposed to being fixed. In his proposal for understanding self-construction, self-narratives are typically driven by some kind of acknowledged trouble or something that is being jeopardized. One of the cornerstones of his theory on selfhood is that self is constructed through interaction with the world as a product of transaction and discourse (Bruner, 1997, p. 146). These interactions involve what Bruner describes as a mix of *outer knowledge* (coming from other people's statements) and *inner knowledge* (self-knowledge) about ourselves, which is generated through our encounters with events and circumstances in the world (Bruner, 1997, p. 147). Furthermore, and as mentioned earlier, our encounters with the world are not fixed, but products of our abilities to construct meaning not only on our own, but in interaction with the world. Following this line of theorizing, Jenkins (2008) argued that our identity as persons rests upon a dialectic process where we present ourselves to others, who in response may affirm or challenge identities we present. The responses of others provide feedback to us, which we then accept or reject and integrate as part of how we see ourselves and this process takes place through the use of reflective thinking (Jenkins, 2008). This is also in line with Bruner's theorizing where he suggested a whole list of indicators or cues of selfhood, and which also are the components seen in narratives (e. g. agency, social reference, evaluation, reflective qualia, positional indicators) (Bruner, 1997, p. 149).

Perhaps one the most central concepts in Bruner's theorizing of the self and identity, and also a concept of importance for understanding identity construction, is the concept of agency. "Agency indicators refer to acts of free choice, to voluntary actions, and to initiatives freely undertaken in pursuit of a goal. They are legion, ranging from signs of mere hesitation to expressions of intentions" (Bruner, 1997, p. 149). Coming from cultural cognitive developmental psychology, Bruner also set out to identify the ontogenies of autobiographic memories and its close relation to language. Together with his colleagues, he documented the very early use of self-accounting in the bedtime soliloquies of a two-year-old girl as she went over her daily life experiences (Nelson, 1989). This suggests that narratives serve a regulative purpose from the early onset of children's development.

Identity construction in children with developmental speech and language disorders

Much of the research with children with developmental speech and language disorders has used quantitative measures and has been *on* rather than *with* children. For example, there is evidence to suggest that the quality of life of these children may be compromised (Eadie et al., 2018; Feeney, Desha, Khan, & Ziviani, 2017; Feeney, Desha, Ziviani, & Nicholson, 2012); that they present with low self-esteem (Jerome, Fujiki, Brinton, & James, 2002; Lindsay & Dockrell, 2000; Lindsay, Dockrell, & Palikara, 2010); that they may be at risk for both emotional difficulties (Clair, Forrest, Yew, & Gibson, 2019) and academic difficulties (Stothard, Snowling, Bishop, Chipchase, & Kaplan, 1998). There has been little research *with* children that has explored identity construction.

However, in recent years, the voice of children with disabilities has been foregrounded in research, underpinned by Article 12 of the United Nations Convention on the Rights of the Child (UNCRC, 1989), which states that:

> States Parties shall assure to the child who is capable of forming his or her own view the right to express those viewsfreely in all matters affecting the child, the views of the child being given due weight in accordance with the age and maturity of the child.

Tisdall (2018) also argued that other newerarticles (e.g. Article 23 and Article 7) concerning children with disabilities were less well-known. Furthermore, Tisdall claimed that although the importance of listening to the voices of disabled children has been acknowledged, it is still not well-understood or used in practice. Wickenden (2018) similarly pointed out that although there have been improvements in attitudes to disability, in many low- and middle-income countries, discrimination and exclusion has changed very little.

There has recently been some research on identity construction in children with developmental disabilities and developmental speech and language disorders. For example, Wickenden (2018) reported that when disabled children from low-income countries (i.e. India and Uganda) described themselves, they presented themselves in similar ways to nondisabled children. Wickenden (2018) also found that their disability was not their main focus with regard to identity construction. In a recent study, Lyons and Roulstone (2017) used narrative inquiry, focusing on small stories, of eleven 9–12-year-old Irish children who presented with developmental speech and language disorders. The aim of this study was to generate storied accounts of the children's everyday experiences of growing up in the context of living with developmental speech and language disorders. Each child participated in 5–6 semi-structured interviews over a six-month period. The interviews took place in familiar settings that were chosen by the children and their parents, e.g. clinics, schools, the children's home. After the interviews, the interviewer summarized her understanding of the respective child's multiple identities to ensure that she had understood their intended meanings. Children were invited to comment on or change the stories. The authors used thematic analysis as well as analysis of syntactic markers of agency and evaluative language to interpret the data. Two overarching themes were identified which were reflected in the children's desired identities (e.g. being competent, being good and socially attractive) and undesired identities (being different when assigned labels *by* others and undesired identities assigned *to* others) (Lyons and Roulstone, 2017, p. 510). A specific methodological strength of the study is that it took place over a six-month period which provided opportunities to build relationships with the children and explore identity construction over time, as opposed to "one-off" interviews.

Given that identity construction with children with developmental speech and language disorders is a relatively new field, methods for carrying out research on identity construction with this group of children is still in the early stages. In the following section, we summarize some methodological considerations that have been suggested, challenges one might be faced with, and recommendations for how to support children with developmental speech and language disorders in constructing narrative identity.

Methodological challenges and recommendations when conducting narrative inquiry with young children with language disabilities

It is important that researchers are aware of methodological challenges and decisions when exploring identity construction in children with developmental speech and language disorders. First, given that children with developmental speech and language disorders present with specific difficulties with talking and narrative abilities, this may present challenges to researchers wishing to use narrative inquiry. Conducting narrative inquiry with children with developmental speech and language disorders requires solid knowledge of children's language (dis)abilities, skills on ways of interacting and engaging with children, and knowledge about developmental speech and language disorders. For example, knowledge about language disorders in children is crucial to enable researchers to avoid misinterpretations of intended meanings. Hence, it is important for researchers to consider the role of context, background knowledge, as well as use of props and scaffolds to enable children to tell their stories. For example, it may be useful to use drawings, books, and photographs to facilitate young children to talk about experiences. Children with developmental speech and language disorders may have difficulties with comprehension of language. Therefore, it is important that the interviewer is aware of the complexity of questions and checks that the child has understood the questions. One of the challenges that children with developmental language disorders can struggle with is understanding and producing grammatical tense-markers and temporal markers. This in turn may lead to misunderstandings of the temporal sequence of the narrative. However, contextualizing the child's language in time and space and reflecting on background information may help avoiding misunderstandings.

Based on their recent and pioneering experiences conducting narrative identity interviews with young children, Lyons and Roulstone in a recent paper discuss methodological considerations when using narrative inquiry with young children with developmental speech and language disorders (Lyons & Roulstone, 2018). They argued that narrative inquiry can be used to explore identity construction and well-being in children with developmental speech and language disorders for a number of reasons. First, narrative inquiry can be used in a range of ways and they argued that the use of a conversational definition of narrative, as described by Ochs and Capps (2001), allowed for the co-construction of data between the interviewer and the child. They also argued that analysis of evaluative dimensions, described by Peterson and McCabe (1992), provided opportunities to explore implicit and explicit meanings (Lyons & Roulstone, 2018, p. 18). They claimed that the units of analysis which suited the 9–12-year-old children in their study were 'small' stories rather than 'big' stories. 'Small stories' provide possibilities for self and identity construction (Goffman, 1959) and are more likely to take place in everyday life experiences (Bamberg & Georgakopoulou, 2008).

Regarding data generation, Lyons and Roulstone (2018) recommended that researchers take time to set up a comfortable context to facilitate children to talk about their experiences. It is important that researchers are flexible and use specific prompts and scaffolding that suit to the needs of each child. Given the heterogenous profile of children with developmental speech and language disorders, techniques for facilitating co-constructed conversational narratives will differ depending on the specific child's age, temperament, and speech/language profile. It is also important that researchers demonstrate rigour and manage potential biases. Following Braun and Clarke (2013) and Christensen (2004), among others, they suggest that the conscious use of reflexivity (critical reflection) throughout the research process is important, which also enhances credibility and trustworthiness (Lyons & Roulstone, 2018, p. 21). In qualitative research with children, it is also important to consider power differences between adults and children. Lyons and Roulstone (2018) recommended involvement of children in aspects of the research process such as giving children opportunities to make decisions during the data-generation process, asking children to select pseudonyms, inviting them to check the transcripts or researcher's interpretation of their stories, ongoing processes to obtain assent making it easy for them to say no if they do not wish to participate in any aspect of the research (see also Rabiee, Sloper, & Beresford, 2005, and Sota, Hartman, & Wilkins, 2006, for ways to involve children with little or no communication).

Voices of young Irish and Danish children growing up with developmental speech and language disorders

In order for the reader to get a better grasp of how narrative inquiry may be used for identity construction with children with a developmental speech and language disorder (LDs), we provide two examples from our own data with Danish and Irish children. In the University Clinic for Developmental Communication Disorders identity construction was explored in a small group setting with two children with LD and conducted by psychology master students in their final year. The therapy sessions were organized around different topics and the following example is from the session with the topic "Friends and Afterschool Activities". In the example a 11-year-old girl with LD clearly tried to express the ways in which she had many thoughts about her own identity as a friend, but at the same time she was being restricted by her language impairment in fully being able to express herself. It also seems that the girl has the desire to position herself as a good friend. The following except illustrates this:

> I: So how would you say you are as a person or a friend?
> C: Well (pause) I am funny, I am friendly, I am helpful, I am … it's difficult to sort of find the right word, what more … (pause) there is something that is called generous. Generous or however you pronounce it.
> I: … so you are a girl whose friends would say she's … she is generous …
> C: I don't quite remember what generous means.
> I: Generous is when one, well treats others well, and wants to do something good for other people.
> C: YES; THAT IS WHAT I AM! That is actually just what I need, like I always think about it, that I want to help other people, but I just didn't quite know that there was a word that was it. And it is that, now I know that that is what it means!

The above example illustrates how the dialogue between the therapist and the girl enforces the girl's abilities to express her thoughts about herself. It is important to mention that the girl had been coming to the clinic for assessment and treatment over a period of nine months and during this period her and the respective therapist had built up a close relationship, so she felt confident with the therapist. During the period of assessment and treatment the girl had often touched upon her role in relationship to her peers at school and was to some extent able to profile herself in a positive way, although it was often unclear how well she herself was able to understand the terminology she used. In many ways it seemed the statements about social competences that the girl used were echoes of how she heard other children surrounding her in school talk about positive peer behaviours, whereas it was unclear how well the girl herself actually understood the meaning of the phrases. It was also clear that the girl felt alone and had difficulties engaging in social activities with peers. It became clear that the girl had a large desire to be like her school peers and longed for social relationships. Compared to the assessment sessions in the clinic the identity construction sessions allowed the girl to reflect in much more depth on her thoughts about herself and gave her confidence to reveal her doubts and weaknesses in understanding herself in relation to others. For most children with LD the feeling of being less knowledgeable about the meaning of words becomes a reality very early in their life. With time this feeling often leads to embarrassment and stigma, which again leads to the children, in order to save face-becoming reluctant to ask for further explanations or assistance. In the case of the girl in our example, she had clearly developed a personal strategy for learning some of the expressions of how one should be to be a good friend, however she had difficulties remembering the words and understanding the meaning of them. During the identity construction sessions, she received help to better understand her own thoughts about herself, to expand her vocabulary for how to express her thoughts, and also the acceptance that being different and asking for help does not mean being abnormal.

As already discussed, Lyons and Roulstone (2017) used narrative inquiry to explore identity construction in 9–12-year-old children presenting with developmental language disorders. One of the participants in this study was Blade, who was an 11-year-old boy who presented with developmental language disorder. Because of his ongoing language difficulties, he was referred to a language class for two years which meant that he had to leave his local school. When he returned to his local school, he received additional support whereby he left the classroom two or three times a week for support with English and mathematics. Blade negotiated his multiple identities in the interviews. His desired identities were that he was competent, socially desirable and good. Receiving additional supports was problematic for Blade because it singled him out from peers, not on his terms, in a visible way and jarred with his desired identity to be "cool". He explicitly rejected undesired identities of "sad" and "special". For example, in this extract from Lyons and

Roulstone (2017, p. 10), Blade rejected an identity of "special" and wanted to fit in like everyone else. Blade was also aware that stigma may be associated with having a developmental speech and language disorder and he referred to shame and exclusion. His use of a negative marker "not" could be interpreted to mean that he believed that children with speech and language disorders *do* feel ashamed and *are* excluded. He argued that children should not feel alone and he explicitly spoke about the importance of hope.

> "Blade", Interview 5
> I: Are you going to get any extra help then in this school Blade?
> P: I don't need extra help. I'm not like a special person, I just, I'm just like the rest of the people in my class …
> [the researcher was clarifying her understanding of what Blade said in previous transcripts]
> I: And the other thing I remember you said, Blade that I remember is, you said it is important not to be ashamed.
> P: And not to be left out.
> I: And not to be left out.
> P: And not to be don't be sad if you think you are the only one that's speech, language, if you have problems, but you don't. You don't have to worry because there will be people you will probably know who exactly have that type of speech. There's a problem with it, so. If I was them I wouldn't be sad. You have to keep your hopes up and it will improve.

Summary and thoughts for the future

Narrative inquiry and identity construction have been used as a window into understanding everyday life experiences of adults with and without disabilities for some decades now. It is only recently that researchers have set out to explore how to use narrative inquiry as a method for understanding the lives of non-disabled and disabled children. Results from the few studies that have been carried out with these children suggest that they present themselves as fitting in, belonging and being like their peers, with communication disability as one aspect of their multiple identities. These pioneering studies have shown that children with developmental speech and language disorders are actively constructing multiple identities and are aware of stigma when identities are "spoiled" (Goffman, 1963). There may be perceived challenges with regard to using narrative inquiry with children with developmental speech and language disorders, who by the nature of their difficulties may find it difficult to participate in *talk* activities and interviews. However, as we have seen in this chapter, having a developmental speech and language disorder does not preclude children from being participants in narrative inquiry studies.

Currently, narrative inquiry is used as a research method, however one could speculate how to expand some of the knowledge and techniques from narrative inquiry into applied tools for practitioners working with children with LDs. As mentioned above, children with LDs are at risk for developing mental health problems (depression, anxiety, low self-esteem, low levels of education, etc.). One could speculate that the child's participation in identity construction activities could have a mediating effect on the child's mental health, and indirectly serve as a protective factor in the child's development. The child's ability to better express how others see and understand it as well as the child's ability to better understand itself could serve to boost the child's self-confidence and self-efficacy.

One might imagine that if practitioners, special education teachers, and psychologists (although, psychologists hardly have time allocated to do anything more than structural testing of the child) became knowledgeable about the techniques used in narrative inquiry (e.g. storytelling) this would facilitate them to discover new ways to incorporate narrating activities in their daily support of the child. In this way an increasing number of children with a LD could perhaps be supported in having a voice, which then could provide them with the strength to better speak up for themselves. Attempts could also be made into piloting methodologies for how to apply narrating in peer groups. These applied activities would, however, require main policy changes and political formations, and long-term national investments.

Acknowledgements

We would like to thank the psychology students (Camilla and Marie) for assistance with the Danish data generation.

References

Acton, C. & Hird, M. (2004). Toward a sociology of stammering. *Sociology*, 38(3), 495–513.

Bamberg, M. & Georgakopoulou, A. (2008). Small stories as a new perspective in narrative and identity analysis. *Text and Talk*, 28(3), 377–396.

Barrow, R. (2011). Shaping practice: The benefits of really attending to the person's story. In R. Fourie (Ed.), *Therapeutic processes for communication disorders: A guide for clinicians and students* (pp. 19–34). Hove: Psychology Press.

Baumeister, R.F. (2005). Self-concept, self-esteem, and identity. In V.J. Derlega, B.A. Winstead, & W.H. Jones (Eds.), *Personality: Contemporary theory and research* (2nd Edition) (pp. 246–280). Belmont: Thomson/Wadsworth.

Bruner, J. (1997). A narrative model of self-construction. *Annals of the New York Academy of Sciences*, 818(1), 145–161.

Burden, R. (2008). Is dyslexia necessarily associated with negative feelings of self-worth? A review and implications for future research. *Dyslexia*, 14, 188–196.

Clair, M.C.S., Forrest, C.L., Yew, S.G.K., & Gibson, J.L. (2019). Early risk factors and emotional difficulties in children at risk of developmental language disorder: A population cohort study. *Journal of Speech, Language, and Hearing Research*, 62(8), 2750–2771. doi:10.1044/2018_JSLHR-L-18-0061.

Eadie, P., Conway, L., Hallenstein, B., Mensah, F., McKean, C., & Reilly, S. (2018). Quality of life in children with developmental language disorder. *International Journal of Language & Communication Disorders*, 53(4), 799–810. doi:10.1111/1460-6984.12385.

Feeney, R., Desha, L., Khan, A., & Ziviani, J. (2017). Contribution of speech and language difficulties to health-related quality-of-life in Australian children: A longitudinal analysis. *International Journal of Speech-Language Pathology*, 19(2), 139–152. doi:10.3109/17549507.2016.1151935.

Feeney, R., Desha, L., Ziviani, J., & Nicholson, J. (2012). Health-related quality-of-life of children with speech and language difficulties: A review of the literature. *International Journal of Speech-Language Pathology*, 14(1), 59–72.

Gee, J.P. (2000). Identity as an analytic lens for research in education. *Review of Research in Education*, 25, 99–125.

Gee, J.P., Allen, A., & Clinton, K. (2001). Language, class, and identity: Teenagers fashioning themselves through language. *Linguistics and Education*, 12(2), 175–194.

Glintborg, C. (2015). Disabled and not normal: Identity construction of adults following an acquired brain injury. *Narrative Inquiry*, 25(1), 1–22.

Goffman, E. (1959). *The presentation of self in everyday life*. New York: Doubleday.

Goffman, E. (1963). *Stigma: Nnotes of the management of spoiled identity*. London: Penguin.

Hiles, D., Čermák, I., & Chrz, V. (2017). Narrative inquiry. In C. Willig & R. Stainton (Eds.), *The Sage handbook of qualitative research in psychology* (pp. 157–175). London: Sage Publications.

Jenkins, R. (2008). *Social identity* (3rd Edition). London: Routledge.

Jerome, A., Fujiki, M., Brinton, B., & James, S. (2002). Self-esteem in children with specific language impairment. *Journal of Speech, Language, and Hearing Research*, 45, 700–714.

Lindsay, G. & Dockrell, J. (2000). The behaviour and self-esteem of children with specific speech and language difficulties. *British Journal of Educational Psychology*, 70, 583–601.

Lindsay, G., Dockrell, J.E., & Palikara, O. (2010). Self-esteem of adolescents with specific language impairment as they move from compulsory education. *International Journal of Language & Communication Disorders*, 45(5), 561–571.

Lyons, R. & Roulstone, S. (2017). Labels, identity and narratives in children with primary speech and language impairments. *International Journal of Speech-Language Pathology*, 5, 503–518. doi:10.1080/17549507.2016.1221455.

Lyons, R. & Roulstone, S. (2018). Listening to the voice of children with developmental speech and language disorders using narrative inquiry: Methodological considerations. *Journal of Communication Disorders*, 72, 16–25. doi:10.1016/j.jcomdis.2018.02.006.

Meadows, S. (2010). *The child as social person*. London: Routledge.

Nelson, K. (1989). *Narratives from the crib*. Cambridge, MA: Harvard University Press.

Ochs, E. & Capps, L. (2001). *Living narrative: Creating lives in everyday storytelling*. Cambridge, MA: Harvard University Press.

Owens, J. (2007). Liberating voices through narrative methods: The case for an interpretive research approach. *Disability & Society*, 22(3), 299–313.

Peterson, C. & McCabe, A. (1992). Parental styles of narrative elicitation: Effect on children's narrative structure and content. *First Language*, 12(36), 299–321.

Rabiee, P., Sloper, P., & Beresford, B. (2005). Doing research with children and young people who do not use speech for communication. *Children & Society*, 19(5), 385–396.

Shadden, B. (2005). Aphasia as identity theft: Theory and practice. *Aphasiology*, 19(3/4/5), 211–223.

Sota, G., Hartman, E., & Wilkins, D. (2006). Exploring the elements of narrative that emerge in the interactions between an 8-year-old child who uses an AAC device and her teacher. *Augmentative and Alternative Communication*, 22(4), 231–241.

Stothard, S., Snowling, M., Bishop, D.V.M., Chipchase, B., & Kaplan, C. (1998). Language impaired preschoolers: A follow-up into adolescents. *Journal of Speech, Language, and Hearing Research*, 41, 407–418.

Strong, K.A. & Shadden, B.B. (2019). The power of story in identity renegotiation: Clinical approaches to supporting persons living with aphasia. *Perspectives of the ASHA Special Interest Groups.* doi:10.1044/2019_PERSP-19-00145.

Tisdall, K.M. (2018). Applying human rights to children's participation in research. In M. Twomey and C. Carroll (Eds.), *Seen and heard: Exploring participation, engagement and voice for children with disabilities* (pp. 17–37). Oxford and New York: Peter Lang.

Tompkins, V. & Jeffrey Farrar, M. (2011). Mother's autobiographical memory and book narratives with children with specific language impairment. *Journal of Communication Disorders*, 44, 1–22.

UNCRC. (1989). *United Nations convention on the rights of the child.* New York: UNICEF. Retrieved from www.unicef.org/crc/.

Wickenden, M. (2018). "I've got lot to say!": A human rights perspective on recognizing the voices of disabled children globally. In M. Twomey and C. Carroll (Eds.), *Seen and heard: Exploring participation, engagement and voice for children with disabilities* (pp. 39–56). Oxford and New York: Peter Lang.

9 Hope in offenders' narratives of Attention Deficit Hyperactivity Disorder (ADHD)

Nichlas Permin Berger and Lars Fynbo

Introduction

This chapter uses life stories from ten socially vulnerable adults interviewed while they were under supervision by the Danish Probation Service. All interviewees have a history of incarceration and are diagnosed with Attention Deficit Hyperactivity Disorder (ADHD). Most of the interviewees received the diagnosis as adults and during their stay in prison, while a few were diagnosed in childhood.

ADHD is a fast-growing diagnosis that traditionally was considered a child-diagnosis but recently has begun to be applied to adults. The Diagnostic and Statistical Manual of Mental Disorders, DSM-5, describes ADHD as a neurodevelopmental disorder involving symptoms of inattention, hyperactivity, and impulsivity, and the specific patterns of behaviour are characterized by difficulties in organizing daily tasks and activities, excessive talking, failure to pay attention to details, concentration difficulties, and difficulty in sitting in various situations.

A pathological psychiatric diagnosis such as ADHD demarcates a difference between "normal" and "abnormal" (Jutel, 2011). Receiving a psychiatric diagnosis may be perceived as definitive and as a kind of verdict about one's life chances and possibilities. An ADHD diagnosis may also cause feelings of ambivalence and doubt as to the reality of ADHD as well as concerns of negative and stigmatizing consequences (Halleröd, Anckarsäter, Råstam, & Scherman, 2015). A diagnosis can lead to re-interpretation of deviant and negative events in individuals' life stories. However, studies of adults diagnosed with ADHD also show that the process of getting a diagnosis can provide individuals with a sense of control and meaning in an otherwise chaotic life. The diagnosis thus provides a new awareness and a name for their potential individual difficulties, and thereby reduces feelings of individual blame (Toner, O'Donoghue, & Houghton, 2006; Young, Bramham, Gray, & Rose, 2008).

Inspired by the analytical framework of anthropologist Cheryl Mattingly, who studied "hope" as an inherently existential practice amongst socially vulnerable and mentally challenged people (Mattingly, 2010), this chapter investigates how socially vulnerable adult criminals perceive being diagnosed with ADHD and how they narrate hope in relation to their diagnosis. Mattingly identifies hope in her interviewees' stories as "a paradoxical temporal practice and a strenuous moral project" (2010, p. 3). In a similar vein, Nielsen (2018) shows how individuals use an ADHD diagnosis for self-evaluation and self-constitution as parts of their "becoming", and how they use their diagnosis as tools for structuring, evaluating, and experimenting with possibilities in a chaotic life full of "differentness" and difficulties.

Hope can be a paradox because it also carries possibilities of despair. As pointed out by Eaves et al. (2016, p. 38), to maintain hope in situations that may seem difficult and hopeless "individuals must navigate multiple contradictions between reality and possibility, embrace cultural notions of what is deemed acceptable to hope for, and be attentive to hopes and concerns of significant others".

In this chapter, we demonstrate the central implications of being diagnosed with ADHD for one of society's most marginalized groups of adults, namely, adult criminals, including how the interviewees relate their diagnosis to hope. The chapter focuses on three narratives that seem to give hope for a better future. We consider symptoms of ADHD as well as the individual stories told by the "patient" as formed by and in specific social contexts, relations, and interactions – i.e. how does being diagnosed with ADHD make a difference to the interviewees' hopefulness? In the data analysis, a great deal of ambivalence and contradictory or incompatible expectations appeared in the stories, when the interviewees pictured their own and their loved ones' future. This indicates a very complex nature of hope as it is both very personal and difficult to describe. Hope is also socially embedded and culturally interpreted, and indeed linked to both broader social and socio-economic processes (e.g. Rose & Novas, 2005).

Hope as narrative practice

We conceive individuals' use of an ADHD-diagnosis in self-narratives as an active identity formation process framed by what is considered culturally and socially legitimate and trustworthy. So, even though the narrators are active and creative when presenting their life narratives, their stories are told through culturally accessible and legitimate narratives. Gubrium and Holstein (2009) call it "narrative practice" when narratives are both seen as being actively constructed and conditioned by the local context. If narratives constitute identities, the formation of identity can be explored in the analysis of how people tell their story and how identity formation occurs between individual biographies and experiences, on the one hand, and societal discourses, narratives, and rationalities on the other. Berger (2015) has shown how embedded discourses of ADHD in the Prison and Probation Service may open up for individual opportunities to draw upon medically and neurobiologically oriented self-narratives. This chapter thus illuminates both the context in which the self-narratives are constructed, the social function they serve, and the many experiences conveyed through the narratives.

Following Mattingly's (2010) concept of "narrative phenomenology of practice" we look at stories as being actively constructed by drawing on existing cultural resources when people tell their life story, or rather when their life-in-process as narratives unfold in interviews. We attend to how the interviewees use "hope" in their stories to actively construct stronger and more prosperous selves. Mattingly writes that practice of hope is "contested, dynamic and hybrid" (2010, p. 39), meaning that structural theories do not have the ability to capture the complex, everyday reality and the "space of possibility", which is necessary when examining lived experience and social worlds. As Mattingly puts it, it is important to acknowledge that: "Ordinary people can and do still act, even in their ordinary contexts. They sometimes do struggle to remake lives in the most remarkable barren 'social circumstances'. And sometimes these struggles make a difference" (Mattingly, 2010, p. 40).

Below we will look at the discursive role of the ADHD diagnosis in people's sense-making of past events in life as well as in formulated ideas of how future actions will be assessed and how such actions are informed by potential future stories. Described from the point of view of the interviewees, we will provide a picture of the three narratives that are performed in their life stories and the meaning of the ADHD diagnosis. Second, we will show how the ADHD diagnosis plays a role in creating spaces of "hope" (Mattingly, 2010) that connect the personal and the local with larger structural and institutional frameworks, when the interviewees draw on cultural resources to "interpret what sorts of stories they are in and to imagine what sort of stories they might be able to create" (Mattingly, 2010, p. 218).

Interviewing and data

Ten interviews were conducted in the interviewees' private homes during a period in which they were under supervision by the Probation Service and frequently received visits from social workers. Most of the interviewees had served more than one prison sentence. Their experiences with criminal justice institutions differed significantly, as did their criminal histories. Their prison sentences ranged from conditional to long-term unconditional sentences. Some had been convicted for theft, illegal possession of weapons or drug peddling, while others had been convicted for violence and manslaughter. Furthermore, most of the interviewees talked about addiction to alcohol and other drugs.

The empirical data analysed for this chapter consist of interviews with nine men and one woman. They were between 18 and 50 years old. The interviewees were all recruited through frontline workers in the Probation Service. Quotes are not taken from every single interview. For illustrative purposes, we have selected quotes that emphasize key points in data (see also Berger, 2015).

ADHD narratives

The interviewees generally described their past and especially their youth as rather chaotic and fragmented. They told of their involvement in various kinds of criminal activity and their former sense of belonging to such networks, and of violence, substance and alcohol abuse. Many reported upbringings in dysfunctional families characterized by abuse, being bullied in school, feelings of social deviation, and, generally, living life "the rough way", as one interviewee put it. All interviewees started out their criminal activities as adolescents and together with peers, conducting petty crimes such as shoplifting, theft, and drug dealings within their own social network. From there, all interviewees sooner or later moved on to more severe types of crime.

The types of self-narratives identified for this chapter all concern the interviewees' experiences of feeling different during childhood and adolescence and of not being recognized by their social environment. Furthermore, the interviewees generally described ADHD as a chronic and neurobiological condition that they have had all their life, but which has not been recognized until they were adults. Explicit plots regarding the relationship between specific acts of crime and ADHD are not present in the data. The interviewees tend to refer to their crimes as a background or living condition, while using the ADHD diagnosis to exonerate themselves from their criminal acts. Similarly, failure to take responsibility for one's own actions is described as the result of neurological dysfunction. All this supports the chapter's argument that the interviewees draw on culturally embedded narratives of ADHD.

In the following section, we will present the three narratives identified in the data. We will focus on how hope in their stories is initiated and fostered by past events and the presence of specific persons in these narratives.

In the first three sections, we present three different and pervasive types of narratives in the life stories of the criminal interviewees. In the first, "ADHD is my biological destiny", we will show how hope is created in specific biomedical discursive practices that are highly supported by parents, wives, and peers, and by the professional discourse of active citizenship in the prison and probation service (Berger & Eskelinen, 2016; Raitakari & Berger, 2016). In the second, "I would not have been without ADHD", the interviewees identify with ADHD (Berger, 2015). In the third narrative, "My ADHD should have been discovered earlier in my life", the interviewees criticize the school, their parents, and the social system for being irresponsible.

ADHD is my biological destiny

The first narrative stems from a biomedical discourse with an understanding of ADHD as being a neurobiological disease in which the interviewees relate the personal relief and redemption that they experienced when they received the diagnosis. None of the interviewees expressed any suspicion that the diagnosis was wrong or raised questions regarding the actual existence of

ADHD. On the contrary, the ADHD diagnosis confirmed their own as well as others' life-long suspicions that something was wrong with them. The ADHD diagnosis seems to provide them with a legitimate conception of their social deviations; that is, an understanding of why other people during their life rarely understood them, their needs, or their difficulties. Somehow, the fact that they have repeatedly committed crimes also seems to confirm them in the view that their ADHD diagnosis is valid. The interviewees never condemned ADHD as a valid diagnosis or dissociated themselves form the diagnosis. Instead, they appeared to conceive of ADHD as something inherent in their brain "just waiting to be discovered". It is characteristic of all the interviewees that they draw upon a neurological discourse (Rose & Abi-Rached, 2013; Singh, 2013) when talking about ADHD in relation to narrating their past experiences and deviant behaviour. The interviewees seem to translate such life events and their experiences of feeling different into ADHD, which is supported, as they explain, by their need for medicine and its positive effects. For example, when asked what ADHD meant to him, John, who received the diagnosis when he was in his thirties, replied:

> John: I think it is the one thing gives some calm in my life, and that they have recognized that they can actually see that I had it. Because it was difficult that they weren't willing to see it.
> Researcher: The Probation Service?
> John: Yes, them too. I mean, people around me could see that I was going full speed ahead. And they thought it was too bad that someone didn't say "you really need to wake up!" Until [name of his wife] said, "I won't put up with it anymore", so, uhm, then I said, "so come with me, then. I need to talk to the head psychiatrist at [name of the psychiatric hospital ward], when he was there, right? Uhm … then she said, 'Now, they better listen to what I say as well, I'm the one living with you and your family, aren't I?'"

John's account represents an example of how receiving the ADHD diagnosis was a welcome relief. The psychiatrist became the problem solver, as John was given permission to be ill (Jutel, 2011) and John appreciated that people around him could be provided with a rational explanation for his (former) irrational behaviour. He may be referring to ADHD medication when he states that something made his life calmer. He may also, though in a less concrete sense, be referring to the diagnosis itself as the thing that provided John and his family with a meaningful framework for interpreting his excessively extrovert behaviour and troubled life path. ADHD appears as a highly meaningful category for interpreting his problems and behaviour, illustrating that ADHD can have a strong social validity. Receiving the ADHD diagnosis was not questioned in any of the cases, whether it was for the better or not.

By understanding himself as almost destined by biology, John does not, however, seem to give everything up and slide into indifference or biological fatalism. Nor does he sink into resignation and passivity, which would support an identity of a "persister" in terms of crime. Instead, he accepts ADHD as a matter of fact and expresses that now he can actually do something about his life situation that he was not capable of before he received his diagnosis.

In the quote below, Jesper explains how things went when he was diagnosed three or four years earlier as an adult in his mid-twenties:

> Researcher: How did it come about?
> Jesper: Because I went to a psychiatrist [psychiatrist's name omitted] and had it identified there. I went there a few years ago because of my suicidal thoughts and other stuff. Then I dropped out of treatment and then I got that shit again. Then I got there and found out that I had ADHD and some mental problems, as well. Since I got help from him, things have moved forward. I haven't taken any drugs or anything since.
> Researcher: How many years ago is that?
> Jesper: It's about two or three years. I've stayed away from drugs ever since.
> Researcher: Do you take any medication for ADHD?
> Jesper: Yes, I do. I take medicine every day.
> Researcher: So it was really that way around, that there were some other urgent things that made you feel bad? Then you saw that as a way out?
> Jesper: Yes, but I took drugs, because when I took drugs, I was able to calm down and relax, and I felt good about myself and everything. It was like you didn't feel like that, when you were running out of drugs. Then I became really anxious and just had to go out and do everything possible to get money to buy them [the drugs].
> Researcher: Yes, to finance it?
> Jesper: Yes, in fact, a lot of the crime I committed was simply because of that. It was like my job was to make money to support my habit. And when that is your job you really have to perform at a high level every seven days of the week.

Jesper is currently medicated for ADHD and has been so for the past few years. In the quote, ADHD also becomes a moral category, which he uses to legitimize his past drug abuse through an indirect reference to "self-medication". In this way, he makes a symbolic distance with reference to ADHD, where he differentiates himself from a "drug addict" and a "criminal", both of which are typically seen as morally inferior and highly stigmatizing identity categories. He says he used to take many drugs in the past to deal with the fact that he was feeling bad, because of what he later confirmed, namely the existence of ADHD and "some mental problems", as he says. The effect of the illegal drugs in combination with the effect of the medication confirms that his brain somehow has a deficit.

The link to crime lies in the fact that Jesper found it necessary to make sure that he felt well and balanced and therefore had to commit crime in order to get the necessary money. His means to achieving mental well-being and balance are presented as legitimate within an expected culturally recognizable horizon of understanding. He may assume to agree predominantly with the interviewer on the significance of the disorder to which the ADHD diagnosis refers and the widespread medical and neurobiological discourse of ADHD, as well as using drugs as self-medication as a fully legitimate way of reasoning.

I would not have been without ADHD

The interviewees also use the ADHD diagnosis to draw a line – or 'symbolic boundary' (Lamont & Molnár, 2002) – between themselves and their former peers in the criminal network. At the same time, nobody explicitly regrets or explicitly distances themselves from former events and courses of action when talking about crime, drugs, and illegal money. They neither seem to regret nor try to hide what happened to the victims of their criminal actions – though they all found it difficult to talk about their victims. The ADHD diagnosis provides a new narrative through which their identity undergoes an identity reconstruction when moving from a highly stigmatized identity as a "criminal" to a less stigmatized category as being "sick". The ADHD diagnosis is thus a tool through which interviewees seek to understand, legitimize, and place parentheses around their past actions instead of neutralizing or distancing themselves from these criminal or deviant actions (Sykes & Matza, 1957).

With the help of their ADHD diagnosis, the interviewees construct themselves as moral and responsible human beings who have lived with a disease that has had a strong impact on their life choices – and criminal activities. They also emphasize that things would have been different if they had been diagnosed earlier. What is common to the stories is that the interviewees express that as human beings they have always been good and moral, by which they all seem to search for evidence for moral agency (Maruna, 2001). The interviewees thereby create a kind of distinction between their criminal actions and their "true" selves, which can be seen as a way of psychologically distancing themselves from crime and other criminals (Maruna, 2001), while at the same time attempting to create good lives and hope for their future, now that they are diagnosed with ADHD (Mattingly, 2013). The interviewees all say that their lives involve a lot of grief and many difficulties. Challenges in life are also closely related to their suffering of ADHD, they say, as the illness has had a very negative impact on their life courses.

At the same time, and this constitutes a paradox of sorts, the interviewees would not have missed many of the experiences they associate with ADHD. While complaining about the consequences of having had to live lives without being properly diagnosed, they also relate ADHD to wild, fast, and sometimes very exciting life events, i.e. in a positive sense. Their narratives thus express a kind of ambivalence towards the meaning of their illness. While their lives with (undiagnosed) ADHD have brought many negative and difficult experiences, there are in retrospect also positive aspects related to the disease. A kind of narrative ambivalence that seems to provide stories of the future as open-ended and as a "space of possibility" (Mattingly, 2010, p. 39). Thus, there is a strong element of ambivalence in their narratives, as their endeavour to "be good" in the future is described as a daily struggle. Recasting the negative or traumatic life experiences as "redemptive suffering" (Maruna, 2001) and as necessary precursors to current and future success, seems to provide them with hope and better prepared for the future.

For example, Simon is disabled and in a wheelchair. He is about 30 years old and has been to prison many times. Initially, Simon says that he has committed both drug crimes and robbery and that he has led a wild and fast life. In the following interview quote Simon shows what ADHD has meant to him and to his criminal activities:

> Researcher: Did ADHD have any impact on the fact that you have committed crime?
> Simon: Uhm, yes, I think … Yes! That is also part of it, because I have not been given any recognition by the doctors and psychiatrists, that they haven't been able to listen to me. So, it's been full speed ahead, something had to happen constantly. I was very restless. I just had to be in control and rush around, and yes, a party guy, right? It also has – what also plays a big role is that it is the time when you were a criminal, yeah? I'm through with that. You might make a lot of money on drugs, but it isn't worth being nicked again. I don't want to go to prison … I value my family, my children and my wife, that's what means something in my life, right? My family, yeah? And then … It doesn't matter if I could make 50 or 100,000. I don't care because it might just be someone saying the wrong thing. And the past hits you, as it often does, unfortunately. Even if it is wrong and they shouldn't judge people that way, and they do. Yes, but if you are known, yes, then you might be inclined again, if I spend a lot of time in those circles, right?

By using the ADHD diagnosis, Simon tells us that he had always been very restless. Simon emphasizes that opting out of this chapter of his life was an active choice on his part, emphasizing his agency, where he eventually managed to get the doctors to listen to him. Simon tells us that he sees his past as meaningful and exciting, but also that there was something else he would rather spend his time on. The ADHD diagnosis thus serves as a relief for him, providing him with an explanation for why his life has gone the way it has. With reference to the ADHD diagnosis, Simon describes himself as a person of moral status and integrity who misses his children and his wife, and as a person who no longer wants to be in the hands of the Prison and Probation Service. With the ADHD diagnosis, Simon is given the opportunity to reconcile himself with his past and to talk about the transition from a wild and criminal life as a young person to a life where family and children are the highest priority. He appears to be getting tired of the wild life and with the phrase "the past hits you" he also says that these lessons have come at a high price. This kind of ambivalence is expressed to varying degrees in the interviewees' self-narratives.

In different ways, the interviewees all construct a balanced narrative and sense of self, where they on the one hand demonstrate to others their vulnerability due to their chaotic and difficult past and marginalized positions, but on the other hand also show their competency in doing things on their own. Such ambivalence is common in the interviews when the interviewees both talk about themselves as highly irrational and irresponsible adolescents and present themselves as family people focused on living responsible lives and caring for their loved ones.

The criminal interviewees use their ADHD diagnosis to present themselves as moral rather than immoral persons but without distancing themselves from their (immoral) actions. Several interviewees state, like Simon, that they would not have been without many of the experiences associated with their lives. At the same time, they all describe how the diagnosis, on the one hand, was an eye-opener for them in understanding themselves – why they were who they were and acted as they did. On the other hand, it is also clear that their diagnosis is central to the negotiation of status and hierarchy, enabling them to position themselves as anything but "criminal". Most of the interviewees, including Simon, have extended periods of incarceration behind them, and in that particular institutional context the diagnosis is a positive resource in the negotiation of social position (Berger, 2015). A prison can be characterized as a "moral space" that symbolically positions inmates as "immoral others" whom you cannot expect to be trustworthy (Ugelvik, 2015). The ADHD diagnosis in the former inmates' self-narratives opens up a "space of possibility" from which to work on hope. Furthermore, the diagnosis allows the interviewees to reason convincingly to an audience about what to do in their life based on their past, and to explain why their lives have gone in that specific direction as well to draw conclusions about who is to blame.

My ADHD should have been discovered earlier in my life

In this narrative, the environment is held responsible for not having been able to discover their suffering due to ADHD. The interviewees feel that they have been left alone with difficult problems and never been fully accepted by their social surroundings. Furthermore, when engaging with social institutions the interviewees feel that they are not recognized as individuals with mental challenges but rather as challenging individuals. The interviewees thus present themselves as life-long victims of the social welfare system because their ADHD disorder remained undiagnosed for a long time, and they blame the welfare state professionals for failing to recognize "their ADHD", which, for instance, resulted in their lack of learning in school. With a concept proposed by Mattingly, the interviewees thus provide an "indigenous hermeneutics of critique" of the welfare society (Mattingly, 2014). The interviewees talk about not receiving enough help and support to avoid getting into trouble, almost claiming that the welfare state professionals did not offer them any alternatives to crime. In this way, the interviewees transfer the responsibility for their criminal actions to the professionals through the diagnosis. The interviewees state that the professionals (schoolteachers, frontline workers from the municipality and in prison) were often disinterested in their problems and did not offer them much support. The interviewees claim that had they received the diagnosis earlier in life, their lives would have been a lot less complicated. They thus blame the authorities for not having identified their disorder in due time. This type of blaming is common in the data.

When asked about how Carsten, as a child, could have been treated differently by the professionals in the system, Carsten replies:

> Carsten: The problem is that it should have been diagnosed earlier! If it gets discovered, as it does now that they are tested from primary school onwards, to see if they can keep up in school, then you find out if they get left behind a lot. So they soon find out. Today, they are better at discovering it. If you went to school today, then you would have learned it. Today, they have a completely different way of doing things.

Several other interviewees criticize the welfare system's lack of awareness and responsibility while using their criticism to voice an "ethical reflection" (Mattingly, 2013, p. 305). The interviewees thereby create a space in which they are able to problematize their lives in a creative and potentially transformative mode of self-making. The interviewees explicitly identify with former criminals, but at the same time do not condemn or express shame for what they have done.

The ADHD diagnosis casts their life experiences in a new and insightful light and makes them reflect on how their lives would have unfolded if "their ADHD" had been identified earlier in life. Claus, who is somewhere in his twenties, tells about his experience with school and his teachers. His use of the ADHD diagnosis can be seen as a way in which the responsibility for his situation is directed at the conditions while he was growing up and the environment in a broad sense. In the next quote, Claus tells about his upbringing:

> Researcher: And how old are you now?
> Claus: I'm [somewhere in his twenties]. But I could see it [ADHD] when I saw it on paper and read about it. And looking back at my behaviour patterns and so on, I can't understand why it [his ADHD] wasn't identified earlier. I went to the school psychologist when I attended preschool, because I was fighting a lot. Back then, it wasn't that known, they didn't know anything about it [ADHD]. So she [the preschool teacher] just said it was because of my parents' divorce. Then I was thrown out of school and got into abuse and things like that, and then we didn't even start it [to find out what was wrong].

> Researcher: And it was back in primary school that you became aware that something was wrong?
> Claus: Yes, even back then I had my behaviour. They didn't put a name on it until several years later. Looking back, I can't understand why they didn't discover it [the ADHD]. She is a psychologist, so why did she not discover it or consider it. But she didn't.

In the quote above, Claus blames and criticizes the professionals at his school for not have done more for him, and he further clarifies this by saying that they should have discovered "it", i.e. the ADHD. He compares school today and back then, saying that if it was today, his ADHD would have been identified a lot earlier, maintaining that he would have avoided many of the negative experiences in his life, had this been the case. He was bullied by peers, for which he blames both the school, his parents, and the welfare system.

Discussion

The chapter has demonstrated how the appearance of ADHD in self-narratives of individuals in rather marginalized positions may be able to create hope, optimism, and restore moral agency. We have demonstrated how being given the diagnosis of ADHD affects the formerly incarcerated interviewees' attempts to evaluate (and narratively construct) their life courses from a more hopeful perspective than they possibly could do before receiving their diagnosis. The interviewees do this by presenting themselves as moral human beings who have a psychiatric disorder, which when left undetected and untreated may cause them to perform immoral actions. With the coming of the diagnosis comes new opportunities of narrating a new moral self without having to neutralize former criminal actions. While dividing their selves between a self before the diagnosis and a self after the diagnosis, the interviewees maintain – at least to a certain degree – an understanding of their own life course as a continuous, coherent, and meaningful process. In doing this, the interviewees use their diagnosis as a tool of hope, enabling them to remain optimistic about their future and, more generally, their lives. What we suggest here is not hope as "blind optimism" or as "romance of desistance" (Mattingly, 2010, p. 233). Rather, we suggest conceiving the former inmates' self-narratives as struggles to maintain and "cultivate" hope in creative ways by drawing upon popular narratives of ADHD.

Thus, the ADHD diagnosis does not primarily stigmatize the interviewees. Instead, the diagnosis provides them with hope and a way of explaining their immoral activities and social deviations, while enabling them to conceive of themselves as responsible persons who, for example, care for their families and friends.

Incorporating the ADHD diagnosis into their self-narratives allows them to create a story about themselves that is well-known and validated by contemporary therapeutic knowledge. It is also an example of the medicalization of everyday life. The interviewees seem to expect that by referring to ADHD they will subsequently be perceived as not being morally deviant (McAdams, 2008; Presser, 2009) and gain moral sympathy and recognition from the interviewer (Furedi, 2004, p. 173).

The popular and culturally embedded narratives of ADHD, which are part of the self-narratives, primarily draw on biomedical and neurobiological discourses in which the brain is the core of the ADHD disorder.

ADHD allows the interviewees to create credible and culturally legitimate self-narratives, where social problems and past events are closely linked to ADHD. The self-narratives draw on a biomedical understanding of ADHD, in which ADHD is seen as a chronic defect in the brain and the interviewees connect the existence of ADHD to their personal destiny. This particular narrative is pervasive throughout the data material.

Destiny is expressed in the narrative "My ADHD should have been discovered earlier in my life", where the system as a whole, welfare state professionals, and the person's family are strongly criticized for not being sufficiently attentive, helpful, and timely. As an ethical reflection this narrative opens up the possibility of redefining the narrative of oneself from being a "criminal" to being "sick" as a moral journey, where they try to do some good. The interviewees make use of crime-reducing "narratives of desistance" (Maruna, 2001) that facilitate new self-understandings and identities as prosperous and non-criminal (Berger, 2015). From the interviews, we can see that the interviewees construct a "redemption script" (Maruna, 2001) using the ADHD diagnosis, which transforms a pattern of deviance and problems into a seemingly meaningful life, providing a sense of direction and hope. Although their use of the three narratives tended to vary, the main story was the same. As Maruna points out, people who can successfully tell a redemption story about themselves can resist damage from stigmatization, "repair" their identities, and have greater agency to act in generative and prosocial ways (2001).

When an ADHD-diagnosis is integrated into individuals' self-narratives, the diagnosis becomes a kind of prism through which it is possible to understand and explain themselves to other people. The interviewees relate their ADHD diagnosis, their experiences of feeling different throughout their lives, being socially isolated and not feeling understood, and having many problems in school. This is in line with other studies of adults' experiences of being diagnosed with ADHD (for example, Young et al., 2008). The diagnosis thus seems to provide such a strong and meaningful explanatory framework that it can frame the entire life of people's stories about themselves. At the same time, there is generally a strong acceptance of, as well as an absence of criticism of, the ADHD diagnosis and its timeliness, which differs from studies among other groups of people diagnosed with ADHD.

References

Berger, N.P. (2015). The creative use of the ADHD diagnosis in probationers' self-narratives. *Journal of Scandinavian Studies in Criminology and Crime Prevention*, 16 (1), 122–139.

Berger, N.P. & Eskelinen, L. (2016). Negotiation of user identity and responsibility at a prerelease conference. *Qualitative Social Work*, 15(1), 86–102.

Eaves, E., Nichter, M., & Ritenbaugh, C. (2016). Ways of hoping: Navigating the paradox of hope and despair in chronic pain. *Culture, Medicine, and Psychiatry*, 40 (1), 35–58.

Furedi, F. (2004). *Therapy culture: Cultivating vulnerability in an uncertain age.* London: Routledge.

Gubrium, J.F. & Holstein, J.A. (2009). *Analyzing narrative reality.* Thousand Oaks: Sage.

Halleröd, S.L.H., Anckarsäter, H., Råstam, M., & Scherman, M.H. (2015). Experienced consequences of being diagnosed with ADHD as an adult: A qualitative study. *BMC Psychiatry*, 15(1), 410–431.

Jutel, A.G. (2011). *Putting a name to it: Diagnosis in contemporary society.* Baltimore: The Johns Hopkins University Press.

Lamont, M. & Molnár, V. (2002). The study of boundaries in social sciences. *Annual Review of Sociology*, 28, 167–195.

McAdams, D.P. (2008). Personal narratives and the life story. In O. John, R. Robins, & L.A. Pervin (Eds.), *Handbook of personality: Theory and research* (pp. 242–262). New York: Guilford Press.

Maruna, S. (2001). *Making good: How ex-convicts reform and reclaim their lives.* Washington, DC: American Psychological Association.

Mattingly, C. (2010). *The paradox of hope: Journeys through a clinical borderland.* Berkeley: University of California Press.

Mattingly, C. (2013). Moral selves and moral scenes: Narrative experiments in everyday life. *Ethnos*, 78(3), 301–327.

Mattingly, C. (2014). *Moral laboratories: Family peril and the struggle for a good life.* Berkeley: University of California Press.

Nielsen, M. (2018). Structuring the self: Moral implications of getting an ADHD diagnosis. *Ethnos*, 83(5), 892–908. doi:10.1080/00141844.2017.1362454.

Presser, L. (2009). The narratives of offenders. *Theoretical Criminology*, 13, 177–200.

Raitakari, S. & Berger, N.P. (2016). Making active citizens in the community in client-worker interaction. In Kirsi Juhila, Suvi Raitakari, & Christopher Hall (Eds.), *Responsibilisation at the margins of welfare* (pp. 106–127). London: Routledge.

Rose, N. & Abi-Rached, J.M. (2013). *Neuro: The new brain sciences and the management of the mind.* Princeton: Princeton University Press.

Rose, N. & Novas, C. (2005). Biological citizenship. In A. Ong & S.J. Collier (Eds.), *Global assemblages: Technology, politics, and ethics as anthropological problems.* Malden: Blackwell.

Singh, I. (2013). Brain talk: Power and negotiation in children's discourse about self, brain and behaviour. *Sociology of Health & Illness*, 35, 813–827.

Sykes, O. & Matza, D. (1957). Techniques of neutralization: A theory of delinquency. *American Sociological Review*, 22(6), 664–670.

Toner, M., O'Donoghue, T., & Houghton, S. (2006). Living in chaos and striving for control: How adults with attention deficit hyperactivity disorder deal with their disorder. *International Journal of Disability, Development and Education*, 53(2), 247–261.

Ugelvik, T. (2015). The rapist and the proper criminal: The exclusion of immoral others as narrative work on the self. In *Narrative criminology: Understanding stories of crime* (pp. 23–41). New York: New York University Press.

Young, S., Bramham, J., Gray, K., & Rose, E. (2008). The experience of receiving a diagnosis and treatment of ADHD in adulthood: A qualitative study of clinically referred patients using interpretative phenomenological analysis. *Journal of Attention Disorder*, 11(4), 493–503.

10 Conclusion and future perspectives

Chalotte Glintborg and Manuel L. de la Mata

Once diagnosed with a disability, there is a risk that this label can take a master status in terms of not only a person's identity, but a whole family's identity. Reification of the diagnosis can be oppressive because it subjugates humanity such that everything a person does can be interpreted as part of the disability. This book has investigated how being diagnosed with various disabilities impacts on identity and how narratives can play a vital role in identity construction. The majority of chapters focus on cognitive disabilities, since subjective experiences from persons with neurological or mental impairments have rarely been seen as reliable or as important sources for information (e.g. Gracey et al., 2008). Such a view on cognitive impairments draws on cognition-based ableism that produces a logic in which the lack of particular cognitive abilities can serve as a justification for the denial of human rights (Wolbring, 2008). For instance, some people with cognitive impairments may have their choices and freedoms taken away without consultation, as they are deemed unable to understand the potential consequences of their actions (Hollomotz, 2014). In addition, there is a risk of not being believed when you have a cognitive impairment. This risk can be even greater with a communication disability without the capacity to narrate and, thus, stand up for yourself.

Therefore, the aim of this book was to amplify voices that may have otherwise remained silent and to utilize storytelling as a way of communicating the participants' realities to a larger and more in-depth understanding of the participants' points of view. Moreover, to unfold the possibilities in narrative inquiry. The knowledge gained in this book offers the reader a deeper understanding of the subject material and extra insight to apply the stories to their own context.

Across the chapters, we see how narratives can play different roles. Moreover, how different scaffolding means to narrate can play a vital role in compensating cognitive and linguistic impairments.

Before our journey through a wide range of "narratives of disability", Chapters 1 and 2 provide an overall introduction to the book and a more detailed explanation of the notions of identity that serve as a theoretical introduction to the following chapters.

Chapter 3 show that, because of the multimodality, the online literacy practices provide an opportunity for the participants to express their stories of self in a more elaborate way than in offline settings. When communicating through for instance Facebook, Instagram, or e-mail, the wide range of modalities (such as the possibility to post photos, videos, illustrations, or emoticons, or to press a like-button) provides an opportunity to choose tools that compensate some of the difficulties of each individual. Whether a person with aphasia wants to tell a story of self which include the linguistic difficulties or not, they may find ways to do so when being involved in multimodal online literacy practices.

In Chapter 5, Hydén and Forsblad argued that persons living with dementia, together with their relatives and others, can attempt to compensate for the diminishing resources available for presenting and negotiating a narrative identity. Moreover, they revealed the various ways co-constructors and the physical environment can scaffold the narrative. In some cases, it is also possible to see that scaffolds work as vehicles of thoughts. For instance, photographs can, when depicting a situation, be tangible in such a way that they tell parts of the story that the person with Alzheimer's Dementia struggles with and therefore make the story more coherent than what it would have been without the photographs. Other people can also work as vehicles of thought when telling parts of a story for the person with dementia. Thus, it is possible to overcome the challenges that are part of interactional storytelling when having a dementia disease by adopting resources that are available in the brain, in the social surrounding, and the cultural world.

In Chapter 4, Glintborg and Thøgersen illustrated the conflict between a medical and a spiritual discourse. Moreover, which narrative is to be taken as the truth in rehabilitation. Because of the enormous power in professional–survivor relations, there is a risk that the professional's interpretations and narratives about a person with acquired brain injury (ABI) can become the truth and the narratives of persons with ABI or the relative can be silenced. The aim of this chapter was to give voice to couple's narratives of spirituality, beliefs, and post-traumatic growth after illness.

Traditionally, research has focused on the negative consequences of ABI. However, the fact that a substantial proportion of people with ABI do not develop psychological distress means that positive and protective mechanisms are also worthy of consideration. Over the past decade there has been an increase in people subscribing to the idea that positive growth may be possible after ABI, particularly when changes occur in relation to a person's sense of meaning, purpose, heightened spirituality, and enhanced relationships after brain injury. The chapter concludes that dyadic coping in couples contributes to a sense of "we-ness" and promotes strategies to respond to the stressful event caused by illness and, thus, post-traumatic growth. Such strategies can be choosing a positive mindset, spirituality, and creating positive illness narratives. Consequently, research in ABI would be enhanced by incorporation of the relatively new concept of "post-traumatic growth", not least because it offers a psychologically grounded entrée into the area of spirituality in ABI survivors and partners.

In Chapter 6, Saavedra explores the relationship between narratives and illness (and, especially, mental illness). Since illness always entails a break between the self and the world, the function of narratives is to justify or make understandable some specific experience (illness, in this case) within the community. Moreover, in narratives we can examine the narrator's agency both within the narrative (how the narrator describes his/her capacity of acting in the world) and in the way s/he uses the narrative to take control of the experience. Starting from this perspective, Saavedra describes different types of narratives related to illness in different disciplines, including literature. Among them, he focuses on what Falconer calls "Katabatic narratives". The term Katabasis refers to the descent to the underworld of the heroes of the Ancient Greece and is used as a metaphor of the journey to mental illness.

For Saavedra, Katabatic narratives contrasts to "Anabatic narratives" or "recovery narratives". Recovery narratives are another genre fostered by the recovery movement in Anglo-Saxon countries. These narratives are characterized by individual authorship, agency of the narrator (the person with mental illness), upward trajectory, goal-directedness (to make sense the episodes of illness), emotional nature (with subjective experience prevailing over rationalization), and moral and political functions. With regard to the last characteristic, an essential aspect of recovery narratives is their capacity to give voice to people with mental illness, to enable them to regain the authorship of their lives. Thus, recovery narratives do not only represent a "scientific" alternative to traditional narratives about illness, but an alternative moral stance about the place of people diagnosed with mental illness in society. This character may allow them to become a model to be applied not only in the area of mental health but for other groups in situations of inequality and risk of social exclusion.

In Chapter 7, Yuste et al. describe another study in which people with aphasia are scaffolded to describe themselves in three moments of their lives; before the onset of aphasia (past), in the present, and in the future. In this case, the scaffolding is not provided by social networks such as Facebook or Instagram, but by using a qualitative open-ended test, the Twenty Statement Test (TST), which requires to complete sentences starting by the prompt "I am". The TST has been extensively used to document cross-cultural differences in the self. In Yuste et al.'s chapter, although results of the test do not provide self-narratives (but a set of personal or social characteristics or traits and, in general, descriptions of the self), the request of describing the self in three life periods around the onset of aphasia, conceived as a turning point, in McAdams' (2001) terms, may have elicited "quasi-narratives", since a temporal perspective was incorporated. At the same time, the TST may have functioned, in the terminology of sociocultural theory, as a *mediational means*, an artefact that re-mediated identity actions of people with aphasia, facilitating identity reconstruction after the onset of aphasia.

By analysing three different dimensions of the self-description of four participants suffering aphasia after brain stroke, the authors have inquired into how the selves of the participants were reconstructed after aphasia. Interestingly, the less positive self-descriptions were referred to the present, compared not only with their lives before aphasia, but to the future, as well. In the future, the four participants envisioned a more positive view of themselves. Besides the limitations associated to aphasia, they described themselves as better persons. A general reflection may arise from these results, concerning the process of identity reconstruction of the participants. Although the methodology cannot be considered narrative *stricto sensu*, the analysis of the participants' self-descriptions about three life periods may suggest the existence of a plot in their life stories that could have similarities with McAdams' "redemptive self". Further research, using narrative methods, is needed to answer this question.

In Chapter 8, de López Jensen and Lyons focused on how to use narrative inquiry as a method for understanding the lives of disabled children. Moreover, it offered future perspectives on the potentials of narratives as a tool to support the increasing number of children with a language disabilities (LD) to gain a voice, which then could provide them with the strength to better speech up for themselves. Results from the few studies that have been carried out with these children suggest that they present themselves as fitting in, belonging, and being like their peers, with communication disability as one aspect of their multiple identities. These studies have shown that children with developmental speech and language disorders are actively constructing multiple identities and are aware of stigma when identities are "spoiled" (Goffman, 1963). There may be perceived challenges with regard to using narrative inquiry with children with developmental speech and language disorders, who by the nature of their difficulties may find it difficult to participate in *talk* activities and interviews. However, as we have seen in this chapter, having a developmental speech and language disorder does not preclude children from being participants in narrative inquiry studies. It is well known that children with LDs are at risk for developing mental health problems (depression, anxiety, low self-esteem, low levels of education, etc.). The authors suggest that child's participation in identity construction activities could have a mediating effect on the child's mental health, and indirectly serve as a protective factor in the child's development. The child's ability to better express how others see and understand it as well as the child's ability to better understand itself could serve to boost the child's self-confidence. Furthermore, they propose the suggestion, that if practitioners, special education teachers, and psychologists became knowledgeable about the techniques used in narrative inquiry (e.g. storytelling) this would facilitate them to discover new ways to incorporate narrating activities in their daily support of the child. In this way an increasing number of children with a LD could perhaps be supported in having voice, which then could provide them with the strength to better speak up for themselves. Attempts could also be made into piloting methodologies for how to apply narrating in peer groups. These applied activities would however require main policy changes and political formations, and long-term national investments.

Chapter 9 demonstrated how the appearance of ADHD in self-narratives of individuals in rather marginalized positions may be able to create hope, optimism, and restore moral agency. Berger and Fynbo demonstrated how being given the diagnosis of ADHD affects the formerly incarcerated interviewees' attempts to evaluate (and narratively construct) their life courses from a more hopeful perspective than they possibly could do before receiving their diagnosis. The interviewees do this by presenting themselves as moral human beings who have a psychiatric disorder, which when left undetected and untreated may cause them to perform immoral actions. With the coming of the diagnosis comes new opportunities of narrating a new moral self without having to neutralize former criminal actions. Incorporating the ADHD diagnosis into their self-narratives allows them to create a story about themselves that is well-known and validated by contemporary therapeutic knowledge. It is also an example of the medicalization of everyday life. The interviewees seem to expect that by referring to ADHD they will subsequently be perceived as not being morally deviant (and gain moral sympathy and recognition from the interviewer). The self-narratives draw on a bio-medical understanding of ADHD, in which ADHD is seen as a chronic defect in the brain and the interviewees connect the existence of ADHD to their personal destiny. This particular narrative is pervasive throughout the data material. When an ADHD-diagnosis is integrated into individuals' self-narratives, the diagnosis becomes a kind of prism through which it is possible to understand and explain themselves to other people.

Future perspectives

During the 1980s psychologists and sociologists explored the biographical disruptions and reconstitutions that follow serious long-term illness. A growing number of researchers have argued that both identity and self are structured through narrative: a person's identity develops and changes through a constant narrative elaboration and revision that happens in interaction with others (Hydén & Örulv, 2010). Therefore, with reference to a narrative identity approach, an illness brakes the basic narrative threads of a person's life and identity, thus it needs to be reconstructed. However, narrative approaches to understanding the formation and changes of human identity are predominantly used as a theory informing single case studies as a way to unfold a perspective analytically without any further testing or experimentation in terms of its effect and applicability to actually transform or heal disrupted identities.

A future perspective could be to establish the foundations for a new paradigm of identity research that cuts across psychological and cultural research integrating cooperation with health care professionals involved in rehabilitation. As also pointed out by de López Jensen and Lyons in Chapter 8, one could speculate how to expand some of the knowledge and techniques from narrative inquiry into applied tools for practitioners.

References

Goffman, E. (1963). *Stigma: Notes on the management of spoiled identity.* London: Penguin.

Gracey, F., Palmer, S., Rous, B., Psailia, K., Shaw, K., O'Dell, J., et al. (2008). Feeling part of things: Personal construction of self after brain injury. *Neuropsychological Rehabilitation*, 18(5/6), 627–650.

Hollomotz, A. (2014). Are we valuing people's choices now? Restrictions to mundane choices made by adults with learning difficulties. *The British Journal of Social Work*, 44(2), 234–251. https://doi.org/10.1093/bjsw/bcs119.

Hydén, L.C. & Örulv, L. (2010). Interaction and narrative in dementia. In D. Schiffrin, A. De Fina, & A. Nylund (Eds.), *Telling stories: Language, narrative, and social life* (pp. 149–160). Washington, DC: Georgetown University Press.

McAdams, D.P. (2001). The psychology of life stories. *Review of General Psychology*, 5, 100–122. doi:10.1037/1089-2680.5.2.100.

Wolbring, G. (2008). The politics of ableism. *Development*, 51, 252–258. https://doi.org/10.1057/dev.2008.17.

Index

Note: Tables are indexed with bold page numbering.